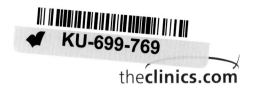

theclinics.com

PEDIATRIC CLINICS
OF NORTH AMERICA

Pediatric Emergencies, Part I

GUEST EDITORS
Donald Van Wie, DO
Ghazala Q. Sharieff, MD
James E. Colletti, MD

February 2006 • Volume 53 • Number 1

SAUNDERS

An Imprint of Elsevier, Inc.
PHILADELPHIA   LONDON   TORONTO   MONTREAL   SYDNEY   TOKYO

W.B. SAUNDERS COMPANY
A Division of Elsevier Inc.

1600 John F. Kennedy Boulevard • Suite 1800 • Philadelphia, Pennsylvania 19103

http://www.theclinics.com

THE PEDIATRIC CLINICS OF NORTH AMERICA	Volume 53, Number 1
February 2006	ISSN 0031-3955
Editor: Carla Holloway	ISBN 1-4160-3539-7

The ideas and opinions expressed in *The Pediatric Clinics of North America* do not necessarily reflect those of the Publisher. The Publisher does not assume any responsibility for any injury and/or damage to persons or property arising out of or related to any use of the material contained in this periodical. The reader is advised to check the appropriate medical literature and the product information currently provided by the manufacturer of each drug to be administered to verify the dosage, the method and duration of administration, or contraindications. It is the responsibility of the treating physician or other health care professional, relying on independent experience and knowledge of the patient, to determine drug dosages and the best treatment for the patient. Mention of any product in this issue should not be construed as endorsement by the contributors, editors, or the Publisher of the product or manufacturers' claims.

The Pediatric Clinics of North America (ISSN 0031-3955) is published bi-monthly by W.B. Saunders, 360 Park Avenue South, New York, NY 10010-1710. Months of publication are February, April, June, August, October, and December. Business and Editorial Offices: 1600 John F. Kennedy Blvd., Suite 1800, Philadelphia, PA 19103-2899. Accounting and Circulation Offices: 6277 Sea Harbor Drive, Orlando, FL 32887-4800. Periodicals postage paid at New York, NY and additional mailing offices. Subscription prices are $125.00 per year (US individuals), $260.00 per year (US institutions), $170.00 per year (Canadian individuals), $340.00 per year (Canadian institutions), $190.00 per year (international individuals), $340.00 per year (international institutions), $65.00 per year (US students), $100.00 per year (Canadian students), and $100.00 per year (foreign students). To receive student/resident rate, orders must be accompanied by name of affiliated institution, date of term, and the signature of program/residency coordinator on institution letterhead. Orders will be billed at individual rate until proof of status is received. Foreign air speed delivery is included in all Clinics subscription prices. All prices are subject to change without notice. POSTMASTER: Send address changes to *The Pediatric Clinics of North America*, Elsevier Periodicals Customer Service, 6277 Sea Harbor Drive, Orlando, FL 32887-4800. **Customer Service: 1-800-654-2452 (US). From outside of the US, call 1-407-345-4000.** E-mail: hhspcs@harcourt.com.

The Pediatric Clinics of North America is also published in Spanish by McGraw-Hill Inter-americana Editores S.A., Mexico City, Mexico; in Portuguese by Reichmann and Affonso Editores, Rua Comandante Coelho 1085, CEP 21250, Rio de Janeiro, Brazil; and in Greek by Althayia SA, Athens, Greece.

The Pediatric Clinics of North America is covered in *Index Medicus, Excerpta Medica, Current Contents, Current Contents/Clinical Medicine, Science Citation Index, ASCA, ISI/BIOMED,* and *BIOSIS.*

Printed in the United States of America.

GUEST EDITORS

DONALD VAN WIE, DO, Division of Emergency Medicine, Department of Surgery, Department of Pediatrics, University of Maryland School of Medicine, Baltimore, Maryland

GHAZALA Q. SHARIEFF, MD, FACEP, FAAEM, FAAP, Associate Clinical Professor, Pediatric Emergency Medicine, Children's Hospital and Health Center/University of California, San Diego; Director, Pediatric Emergency Medicine, Palomar-Pomerado Hospitals, San Diego, California

JAMES E. COLLETTI, MD, Assistant Professor of Emergency Medicine, University of Minnesota School of Medicine; Associate Residency Director, Department of Emergency Medicine, Regions Hospital, St. Paul, Minnesota

CONTRIBUTORS

TONIA BROUSSEAU, DO, Associate Clinical Professor, University of Florida Shands Jacksonville; Attending Physician, Wolfson Children's Hospital, Jacksonville, Florida

SARAH CARSON, MD, Assistant Professor of Emergency Medicine, Department of Emergency Medicine, The University of Arizona, Tucson, Arizona

FORREST T. CLOSSON, MD, Instructor of Pediatrics; Director, Sexual Abuse and Rape Assessment, Division of Emergency Medicine, Department of Pediatrics, University of Maryland Hospital for Children, Baltimore, Maryland

STEPHANIE J. DONIGER, MD, FAAP, Fellow, Pediatric Emergency Medicine, Children's Hospital and Health Center/University of California, San Diego, California

MARK HUDSON, MD, Midwest Children's Resource Center, Children's Hospitals and Clinics of Minnesota, St. Paul, Minnesota

RICH KAPLAN, MSW, MD, Clinical Associate Professor of Pediatrics, University of Minnesota, Minneapolis; Associate Medical Director, Midwest Children's Resource Center, Children's Hospitals and Clinics of Minnesota, St. Paul, Minnesota

KEVIN KILGORE, MD, Assistant Professor of Emergency Medicine, University of Minnesota School of Medicine; Department of Emergency Medicine, Regions Hospital, St. Paul, Minnesota

MAUREEN McCOLLOUGH, MD, MPH, Associate Professor of Clinical Emergency Medicine and Pediatrics, Keck University of Southern California School of Medicine; Director, Pediatric Emergency Department, Los Angeles County–USC Medical Center, Los Angeles, California

GHAZALA Q. SHARIEFF, MD, FACEP, FAAEM, FAAP, Associate Clinical Professor, Pediatric Emergency Medicine, Children's Hospital and Health Center/University of California, San Diego; Director, Pediatric Emergency Medicine, Palomar-Pomerado Hospitals, San Diego, California

GETACHEW TESHOME, MD, Assistant Professor of Pediatrics, Division of Emergency Medicine, Department of Pediatrics, University of Maryland School of Medicine, Baltimore, Maryland

MARY L. THIESSEN, MD, Department of Emergency Medicine, University of Arizona, Tucson, Arizona

DALE P. WOOLRIDGE, MD, PhD, Assistant Professor, Department of Emergency Medicine; Director, Pediatric Emergency Medicine, Department of Emergency Medicine, The University of Arizona, Tucson, Arizona

CONTENTS

Preface   xi
Donald Van Wie, Ghazala Q. Sharieff, and James E. Colletti

Pediatric Minor Closed Head Injury   1
Mary L. Thiessen and Dale P. Woolridge

> Many studies have found conflicting evidence over the use of
> clinical indicators to predict intracranial injury in pediatric mild
> head injury. Although altered mental status, loss of consciousness,
> and abnormal neurologic examination have all been found to be
> more prevalent among head-injured children, studies have observed
> inconsistent results over their specificity and predictive value.
> Children older than 2 years have been evaluated, managed, and
> studied differently than those less than 2 years old. Evidence
> strongly supports a lower threshold to perform a CT scan in younger
> children because they have a higher risk of significant brain injury
> after blunt head trauma.

Clinical Response to Child Abuse   27
Mark Hudson and Rich Kaplan

> This article focuses on current practice in the diagnosis and
> management of the pediatric patient who is a potential victim of
> abuse. We will review diagnostic and management issues in the
> major manifestations of physical and sexual abuse are reviewed.
> This article serves as an aide to practitioners in the recognition of
> and response to child maltreatment.

Pediatric Upper Extremity Injuries   41
Sarah Carson, Dale P. Woolridge, Jim Colletti, and Kevin Kilgore

> The pediatric musculoskeletal system differs greatly from that of
> an adult. Although these differences diminish with age, they present
> unique injury patterns and challenges in the diagnosis and treatment
> of pediatric orthopedic problems.

Newborn Emergencies: The First 30 Days of Life 69
Tonia Brousseau and Ghazala Q. Sharieff

The evaluation and appropriate management of the critically ill
neonate requires knowledge of the physiologic changes and life-
threatening pathologies that may present during this time period.
A broad systematic approach to evaluating the neonate is necessary
to provide a comprehensive yet specific differential diagnosis for a
presenting complaint or symptom. Efficient recognition and prompt
management of illness in the neonatal period may be life saving.
Recently, it has become more important for the emergency department physician to be familiar with the neonate because of early discharge policies. This review provides a systematic approach to the
recognition, emergency stabilization, and management of the more
common newborn emergencies.

Pediatric Dysrhythmias 85
Stephanie J. Doniger and Ghazala Q. Sharieff

Arrhythmias in children are less common than in adults but are
increasing because of successful repair of congenital heart diseases.
Supraventricular tachycardia is the most common symptomatic
pediatric tachyarrhythmia. Atrial flutter and atrial fibrillation in children are attributed largely to structural heart disease. Bradycardia
is defined as a heart rate less than the lower limit of normal for a
child's age, and the most common cause is sinus bradycardia.
Despite the infrequent occurrence of arrhythmias, it is crucial to
expeditiously identify and treat certain rhythm abnormalities
because they can lead to further decompensation.

Abdominal Pain in Children 107
Maureen McCollough and Ghazala Q. Sharieff

Abdominal pain and gastrointestinal symptoms such as vomiting
or diarrhea are common chief complaints in young children who
present in emergency departments. It is the emergency physician's
role to differentiate between a self-limited process such as viral
gastroenteritis or constipation and more life-threatening surgical
emergencies. Considering the difficulties inherent in the pediatric
examination, it is not surprising that appendicitis, intussusception,
or malrotation with volvulus continue to be among the most elusive diagnoses. This article reviews both the self-limited and more
life-threatening gastrointestinal conditions that may present in the
emergency department.

Emergency Medical Treatment and Labor Act: The Basics and Other Medicolegal Concerns   **139**

Getachew Teshome and Forrest T. Closson

The Emergency Medical Treatment and Labor Act (EMTALA) was enacted by Congress because of its concern with an increasing number of reports that hospital emergency rooms were refusing to accept or treat individuals with emergency conditions if the individuals did not have insurance. With increasingly crowded emergency departments and a decreasing number of emergency departments, a periodic review of the effect that EMTALA has on the emergency medical services will prevent unintended consequences of this well-intentioned act.

Index   **157**

FORTHCOMING ISSUES

April 2006
Pediatric Emergencies, Part II
Donald Van Wie, DO,
Ghazala Q. Sharieff, MD, and
James E. Colletti, MD, *Guest Editors*

June 2006
Recent Advances in Clinical Pediatric Urology and Nephrology Practice
Hrair-George O. Mesrobian, MD, and
Cynthia G. Pan, MD, *Guest Editors*

August 2006
Scientific Foundations of Clinical Practice, Part I
Robert M. Kliegman, MD, and
Ellis D. Auner, MD, *Guest Editors*

RECENT ISSUES

December 2005
Diabetes Mellitus in Children
Mark A. Sperling, MD, *Guest Editor*

October 2005
International Adoption: Medical and Developmental Issues
Lisa H. Albers, MD,
Elizabeth D. Barnett, MD,
Jerri Ann Jenista, MD, and
Dana E. Johnson, MD, PhD, *Guest Editors*

August 2005
Pediatric Hospital Medicine
Vincent W. Chiang, MD, and
Lisa B. Zaoutis, MD, *Guest Editors*

PEDIATRIC CLINICS OF NORTH AMERICA FEBRUARY 2006

GOAL STATEMENT

The goal of *Pediatric Clinics of North America* is to keep practicing physicians and residents up to date with current clinical practice in pediatrics by providing timely articles reviewing the state-of-the-art in patient care.

ACCREDITATION

The *Pediatric Clinics of North America* is planned and implemented in accordance with the Essential Areas and Policies of the Accreditation Council for Continuing Medical Education (ACCME) through the joint sponsorship of the University of Virginia School of Medicine and Elsevier. The University of Virginia School of Medicine is accredited by the ACCME to provide continuing medical education for physicians.

The University of Virginia School of Medicine designates this educational activity for a maximum of 90 category 1 credits per year, 15 category 1 credits per issue, toward the AMA Physician's Recognition Award. Each physician should claim only those credits that he/she actually spent in the activity.

The American Medical Association has determined that physicians not licensed in the US who participate in this CME activity are eligible for AMA PRA category 1 credit.

Category 1 credit can be earned by reading the text material, taking the CME examination online at http://www.theclinics.com/home/cme, and completing the evaluation. After taking the test, you will be required to review any and all incorrect answers. Following completion of the test and evaluation, your credit will be awarded and you may print your certificate.

FACULTY DISCLOSURE/CONFLICT OF INTEREST

The University of Virginia School of Medicine, as an ACCME accredited provider, endorses and strives to comply with the Accreditation Council for Continuing Medical Education (ACCME) Standards of Commercial Support, Commonwealth of Virginia statutes, University of Virginia policies and procedures, and associated federal and private regulations and guidelines on the need for disclosure and monitoring of proprietary and financial interests that may affect the scientific integrity and balance of content delivered in continuing medical education activities under our auspices.

The University of Virginia School of Medicine requires that all CME activities accredited through this institution be developed independently and be scientifically rigorous, balanced and objective in the presentation/discussion of its content, theories and practices.

All authors/editors participating in an accredited CME activity are expected to disclose to the readers relevant financial relationships with commercial entities occurring within the past 12 months (such as grants or research support, employee, consultant, stock holder, member of speakers bureau, etc.). The University of Virginia School of Medicine will employ appropriate mechanisms to resolve potential conflicts of interest to maintain the standards of fair and balanced education to the reader. Questions about specific strategies can be directed to the Office of Continuing Medical Education, University of Virginia School of Medicine, Charlottesville, Virginia.

The authors/editors listed below have identified no financial or professional relationships for themselves, their spouse/partner: Tonia Brousseau, DO; Sarah F. Carson, MD; Forrest T. Closson, MD; James Colletti, MD; Stephanie J. Doniger, MD, FAAP; Carla Holloway, Acquisitions Editor; Mark Hudson, MD; Paul T. Ishimine, MD, FACEP, FAAP; Rich Kaplan, MD; Kevin P. Kilgore, MD, FACEP; Maureen McCullough, MD, MPH; Ghazala Q. Sharieff, MD, FACEP, FAAEM, FAAP; Getachew Teshome, MD; Mary L. Thiessen, MD; Donald F. Van Wie Jr., DO; and, Dale P. Woolridge, MD, PhD.

Disclosure of Discussion of Non-FDA Approved Uses for Pharmaceutical and/or Medical Devices: **The University of Virginia School of Medicine, as an ACCME provider, requires that all authors identify and disclose any "off label" uses for pharmaceutical and medical device products. The University of Virginia School of Medicine recommends that each physician fully review all the available data on new products or procedures prior to clinical use.**

TO ENROLL

To enroll in the *Pediatric Clinics of North America* Continuing Medical Education program, call customer service at **1-800-654-2452** or visit us online at www.theclinics.com/home/cme. The CME program is available to subscribers for an additional fee of $195.00.

PEDIATRIC CLINICS

OF NORTH AMERICA

ELSEVIER
SAUNDERS

Pediatr Clin N Am 53 (2006) xi–xiii

Preface

Pediatric Emergencies, Part I

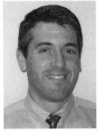   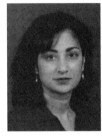   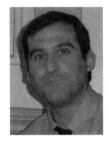

Donald Van Wie, DO   Ghazala Q. Sharieff, MD   James E. Colletti, MD
Guest Editors

According to the Centers for Disease Control and Prevention, there were 113.9 million emergency department visits in 2003, an increase from 95 million visits in 1997. Children account for approximately 25% of these visits. Given the need for quality emergency services for children, pediatric emergency medicine continues to be an important expanding area of medicine. Over the last 20 years significant advances and improvements have occurred in the delivery of emergency care to children which include emergency medicine residency training in pediatric emergencies, pediatric trauma care, pain management for children, pediatric drug dosages, pediatric equipment/supplies in emergency departments and on ambulances, as well as a national poison control system [1]. Even with these great strides, the practice of pediatric emergency medicine continues to evolve. This issue will be the first of two issues of the *Pediatric Clinics of North America* this year that will focus on state-of-the-art information regarding the emergency care of children, adressing current areas of interest, clinical practice, and controversy.

Child abuse remains a frequently encountered possible concern in the emergency department, and having a well thought-out team approach will help ensure the best outcome for the child. Complementing this article on abuse, we also review some of the recent medical legal aspects of pediatric emergency care and provide an update on EMTALA law. Pediatric trauma remains the leading cause of death and disability in childhood. A physician's goal in evaluating head trauma is to accurately identify and diagnose patients who are at risk for serious injury and complications. In the article on pediatric minor closed head injury some of the recent controversies over the use of clinical predictors of intracranial injury are discussed and some proposed decision trees to help guide the management of minor head injury are reviewed. The efficient recognition and prompt management of illness in the neonatal period may be life-saving. In recent years, it has become more important for the ED physician to be familiar with the neonate because of early discharge policies from newborn nurseries. A broad systematic approach is delineated for the reader in the article on newborn emergencies in the pediatric ED. Abdominal pain in children can be difficult to evaluate due to the nonverbal nature of many young children, vague histories, and patient and parental anxiety. This issue of *Pediatric Clinics* will discuss some of the common and most life-threatening causes of abdominal pain in the pediatric age range. The presentation of dysrhythmias can serve as a diagnostic challenge to clinicians because most children present with vague and nonspecific symptoms such as "fussiness" or "difficulty feeding." An update on pediatric dysrythmias is provided because it is critical to identify and appropriately manage these disorders. To round out the issue, upper extremity injuries specific to the pediatric population as well as essential EMTALA and medicolegal concerns are discussed. It is our sincere hope that these updates will be of use for pediatricians, pediatric hospitalists, and pediatric emergency medicine specialists.

We would like to thank all our authors for their time and effort in preparing the manuscripts. We would also like to thank Elsevier and their staff for their support.

Donald Van Wie, DO
*Division of Emergency Medicine, Department of Surgery
and Department of Pediatrics
University of Maryland School of Medicine
110 S. Paca Street, Sixth Floor, Suite 200
Baltimore, MD 21201, USA*
E-mail address: dvanwie@peds.umaryland.edu

Ghazala Q. Sharieff, MD
*Department of Pediatric Emergency Medicine
University of California, San Diego
3030 Children's Way
San Diego, CA 92123, USA*
E-mail address: ghazalaqs@hotmail.com

James E. Colletti, MD
Emergency Medicine Regions Hospital
640 Jackson Street
St. Paul, MN 55101-2502, USA
E-mail address: james.e.colletti@healthpartners.com

Reference

[1] American College of Emergency Physicians. A decade of advancements in pediatric emergency care. Available at: http://www.acep.org. Accessed November 20, 2005.

ELSEVIER
SAUNDERS

Pediatr Clin N Am 53 (2006) 1–26

PEDIATRIC CLINICS
OF NORTH AMERICA

Pediatric Minor Closed Head Injury

Mary L. Thiessen, MD, Dale P. Woolridge, MD, PhD*

*Department of Emergency Medicine, University of Arizona, 1515 North Campbell Avenue,
Tucson, AZ 85724, USA*

Trauma is the leading cause of death and disability in childhood, with approximately 3000 deaths, 50,000 hospitalizations, and 650,000 emergency department (ED) visits per year in the United States [1]. The term concussion has been used interchangeably with mild head injury (MHI) or mild traumatic brain injury (TBI) and has been defined as a trauma-induced alteration in mental status that may or may not involve the loss of consciousness (LOC). Controversy exists over the use of clinical predictors of intracranial injury in pediatric MHI; nevertheless, authors have devised decision trees to help guide the management of minor head injury. Many authors recommend imaging younger children because these children have a higher risk of significant brain injury after blunt head trauma. Neuropsychologic evaluation can detect more subtle changes associated with concussion, and neuroimaging studies may be needed in more severe concussions. Management and return-to-play guidelines have been developed for sports-related concussions of different grades.

Epidemiology

Pediatric MHI comprises a large portion of pediatric trauma cases seen in emergency departments. Among children aged 0 to 14, TBI results in over 400,000 ED visits each year. Injury rates are highest among children 0 to 4. One to two percent of all pediatric patients seen in the ED present with minor head trauma, but only 3% to 5% of those patients have intracranial injury (ICI), and less than 1% of these patients require any neurosurgical intervention [2]. Among recent studies, the incidence of ICI varies from 5% [3] to

---

* Corresponding author.
E-mail address: dale@aemrc.arizona.edu (D.P. Woolridge).

doi:10.1016/j.pcl.2005.09.004   *pediatric.theclinics.com*

25% [4] of neurologically normal children. Over 85% of the 1.5 million TBIs (all ages) occurring annually in the US are considered "mild" [5]. In a recent study of TBI epidemiology of all ages, the average incidence of mild TBI was 503.1 per 100,000 population, with a peak among American Indians/Alaska Natives (1026/100,000 population) and in children younger than 5 years old (1115.2/100,000 population). The mechanisms by which children sustain head injury vary by activity, age, helmet use, and geographic location.

Falls

Many studies of pediatric head injury cite falls as the most common mechanism of injury, ranging from 32% to 91% [6–9]. In a recent epidemiologic study [5] of mild TBI among all ages, the authors found that the mechanism of injury varied considerably by age, with falls frequent at the extremes of age and assaults and motor vehicle trauma in the middle-aged groups. In one retrospective study of children less than 2 years old, 89% of the patients sustained a fall as the mechanism of isolated skull fracture, in which 60% were free falls (from adults arms, tables, beds, bathtubs, and banisters) and 30% were stair falls. Direct falls from heights greater than 3 feet and stair falls are more likely to result in ICI than falls less than 3 feet. However, there is still a 2% to 7% risk of ICI in the infants who fall less than 3 feet [8,10,11]. Although falls may be the most commonly cited mechanism of injury in pediatric head trauma, motor vehicle accidents have been reported to have more significant intracranial pathologies [6].

Infant walkers have remained a threat to child safety when they are not used in safe locations or under close supervision. Thirty-four deaths were reported from infant walker accidents from 1973 to 1999 [12]. Stairs were implicated in 75% to 96% of these accidents. Because of insufficient safety regulations and a high risk of head injuries, the American Academy of Pediatricians (AAP) recommends a ban on the manufacture and sale of mobile infant walkers. The AAP offers stationary play centers as an alternative to mobile walkers [12].

Bicycle helmet legislation has become a strong strategy for head injury prevention among both children and adults. One thousand people die annually from bicycle crashes, and 65% of bicycle-related head injury deaths occur in children less than 15 years old [13]. The Cochrane Collaboration [14] systemic review reported that helmets reduce the risk of head injury up to 88% among cyclists. In a systematic review of five case-controlled trials in which there were 7253 head-injured cyclists (all ages), helmet use was associated with a risk reduction of 65% to 88% from head and brain injury [15].

Pathophysiology of mild head injury

Variations in the definitions of MHI can confuse the way in which patients are classified, evaluated, and treated. The term concussion has been used interchangeably with MHI or mild TBI. If MHI is viewed on an injury severity spectrum, concussion usually refers to milder injuries. The definition used more commonly is by the American Academy of Neurology (AAN): "Concussion is a trauma-induced alteration in mental status that may or may not involve loss of consciousness. Confusion and amnesia are the hallmarks of concussion." [16]. The Head Injury Interdisciplinary Special Interest Group of the American Congress of Rehabilitation Medicine (ACRM) has adopted criteria to help define MHI [17,18]. Further discussion of concussion and mild TBI continues in the sports-related head injury section below.

Head injuries can result from different types of forces. Impact, acceleration–deceleration, and rotational forces directly affecting the head may cause skull and scalp injuries, neural tissue damage, or cerebral vasculature injuries. Brain injury can be subdivided into primary and secondary injuries. Primary brain injury is the result of a direct force to the brain. The severity and location of the primary brain injury dictates the patient's immediate level of consciousness and mental status. Primary brain injury can lead to impaired autoregulation of cerebral blood flow (CBF). Altered CBF regulation, bleeding contusions, and blood–brain-barrier breakdown contribute to brain swelling. Secondary brain injury subsequently results from the traumatic event and multiple interrelated pathophysiologic processes. The loss of consciousness after head injuries, the development of secondary brain damage, and the vulnerability of the brain after an initial insult can be explained by ion fluxes, acute metabolic changes, and CBF alterations [19]. Biochemical mediators involved in secondary brain injury involve excitatory amino acids, free radicals, and opiate peptides [19]. Massive increases in extracellular potassium concentrations can lead to the inhibition of action potentials and ultimately to the loss of consciousness. Sometimes, it may require several seconds or longer for the potassium levels to increase above the threshold level, which can explain the delay to loss of consciousness when an athlete walks off the field and collapses [20]. Delayed brain swelling is a major cause of elevated intracranial pressure, which can lead to brain herniation and death. From minutes to hours after the brain injury, a total-body hypermetabolic state begins, with a marked increase glucose use. However, after the initial phase, cerebral hypometabolism evolves, with decreased protein synthesis and reduced oxidative capacity. Cells are more susceptible to death after a second insult [20]. The final common pathway involves impaired glucose and oxygen delivery to neurons and ultimately neuronal cell death [19].

Children's heads are disproportionately larger in comparison with their body size. Approximately 72% of the adult intracranial volume of 1200 to 1500 mL is achieved by the age of 2 years. The intracranial volume approaches 90% the adult volume by the age of 8 years, and by adolescence, 96% of the volume is achieved. The sphenoid and petrous bones provide a buttress support to pediatric skulls, thus conferring an "architectural advantage" [21]. In addition, the cranial sutures function as joints in infants, allowing for a small degree of movement in response to a mechanical stress [21].

The parietal bone is the skull bone most commonly fractured (approximately 60%–70%), followed by the occipital, frontal, and temporal bones [22]. Fractures are classified as linear, depressed, compound, or basilar. Linear fractures are the most common. In a depressed skull fracture (SF), the bone fragment is depressed below the inner skull table. "Ping-pong" fractures are a special variant of depressed SFs, in which the inner and outer skull table can be dented like a ping-pong ball. These fractures are seen more commonly in a newborn when the cranium is less well mineralized and more prone to distortion. Compound SFs are "open" fractures exposed through the full-thickness scalp laceration. Fractures that have an increased association with inflicted head injury can present as multiple, linear, and complex. These fractures may be comminuted or stellate [23].

The basilar SF is a fracture at the base of the skull involving the temporal or parietal bone. Clinical signs of a basilar SF include CBF rhinorrhea, CSF otorrhea, ecchymosis over the mastoid bone (Battle's sign), periorbital ecchymosis (raccoon eyes), and hemotympanum or cranial nerve seven palsies. Fractures may extend into the petrous portion of the temporal bone and cause tears of the tympanic membrane, disruption of the auditory ossicles, and facial nerve injury [23]. Complications of basilar SFs can lead to permanent hearing loss if the fracture involves the cochlear–vestibular apparatus or facial nerve palsy. CSF fistulas can form as a result of a dural tear in association with a sinus fracture. Undetected CSF fistulas can be source of potential meningitis. The incidence of meningitis in basilar SF ranges from 0.7% to 5%, and in patients who do not have intracranial hemorrhage and Glasgow coma scores (GCS) of 13 to 15, the rate is 1% [22].

Clinical Indicators of intracranial injury

A physician's goal in evaluating head trauma is to accurately identify and diagnose patients who are at risk for serious injury and complications. The management of primary brain injury demands early diagnosis and effective treatment to prevent secondary brain damage. In patients with depressed consciousness or focal neurologic signs, the ICI is easier to diagnose than in fully conscious patients, in whom an evolving ICI can be difficult to recognize [7]. Therefore, it is essential that the risk factors used to predict ICI are reliable. Many of the recommendations that physicians have followed are based on limited data and small study samples. More recent data are now available that involve prospective cohort studies with larger patient populations.

Physicians must determine which patient is at risk for ICI and who would benefit from head CT. Unfortunately, no predetermined set of clinical criteria exist that accurately and reliably predict the presence of ICI. The assessment of the GCS, LOC, mechanism of injury, and neurologic disability can help guide the physician in the evaluation and management. On examination, the physician needs to determine if there has been any change in mental status or other physical parameters from the time of the initial assessment, whether it was carried out by parents or paramedics.

Davis and colleagues [24] suggest that a normal mental status (GCS 15) after an isolated head injury does not warrant a head CT and that the child is not at risk for ICI. A similar suggestion is that only children with LOC, decreased GCS, or SFs should undergo head CT [9]. On the other hand, other studies have shown that historical and clinical factors are poor predictors of ICI. Even children with apparently minor head trauma and normal mental status can suffer ICI [4,25].

Pediatric patients can be difficult to assess clinically in terms of their mental status, behavior, and neurologic function. Therefore, much controversy exists over how to triage, evaluate, and manage these minor head injuries. Abnormal neurologic examination suggestive of ICI have signs and symptoms of headache, vomiting, drowsiness, irritability, amnesia, visual disturbance, focal neurologic signs, dizziness, altered consciousness, or signs of a fractured skull base [7]. An abnormal mental status in pediatric blunt head trauma should be considered if the patient has a GCS less than 15 or if the patient is confused, somnolent, repetitive, or slow to respond to verbal communication [1].

Many studies have attempted to establish clinical predictors of ICI, and although much progress has been gained, controversy still exists surrounding the management of patients with GCS 13 to 15 and brief LOC. A defined set of screening clinical criteria has not been validated or standardized, but many authors suggest clinical predictors of ICI [7,9,26]. The presence of a neurologic deficit is highly suggestive of an ICI [6,7,26,27]. Lloyd and colleagues [7] observed the presence of neurologic abnormalities had greater sensitivity and negative predictive value for ICI than did the presence of a SF. Similarly, Brown and colleagues [11] reviewed head-injured children less than or equal to 10 years old who underwent neurosurgical procedures. Altered mental status was the most common sign or symptom and was identified in 85% of the ICI patients.

Several studies of pediatric head injury have determined clinical predictors of ICI. Quayle and colleagues [27] prospectively studied a cohort of children who had nontrivial head injuries and identified five clinical predictors of ICI (altered mental status, focal neurologic deficit, signs of basilar SF, a SF, and LOC for ≥ 5 minutes). There was also a trend toward an association between seizures and ICI, but it was not statistically significant. Nevertheless, over half of the children with ICI had a normal mental status and no focal abnormalities, two thirds of whom were infants. Taking this into consideration, the authors recommend scanning children who present with the study's five identified clinical predictors as well as children with symptoms such as vomiting, amnesia, LOC, headache, and drowsiness. Although studies have determined independent predictors of ICI, children with ICI may present with subtle signs, especially infants younger than 1 year [27].

Clinical decision rules to predict ICI have been shown to be useful in pediatric populations. Palchak and colleagues [1] preformed an observational cohort investigation of over 2000 children younger than 18 years of age, 62% of whom underwent CT of the head, and found that 7.7% had TBI on CT scans, and 5% had a TBI requiring acute intervention. The study derived a decision rule that demonstrated high sensitivity for TBI and high negative predictive value for identifying children without TBI. The authors combined the data of the two decision trees for recognizing TBI on CT scans and TBI requiring acute intervention (differing only by one clinical predictor). This combined decision tree identified 97 of 98 (99%) children who had TBI on CT, and 105 (100%) children who had TBI requiring acute intervention. The authors conclude that important factors for determining children at low risk for traumatic head injuries include the absence of an abnormal mental status, clinical signs of skull fracture, a history of emesis, scalp hematoma, and headache [1].

A normal mental status or the absence of neurologic deficit does not exclude a serious brain injury. Studies have determined conflicting evidence on the reliability of neurologic signs and symptoms for TBI. Some authors have found that a detailed clinical examination is of no diagnostic value in detecting ICI found on head CT [26,28,29]. This finding has led many practitioners to recommend head CT in patients in whom LOC or amnesia and abnormal mental status are observed as part of the evaluation, to avoid missing an ICI [29]. Several studies have evaluated "most well" pediatric head trauma patients and have determined that neither historical variables (history of seizure, LOC, amnesia, or confusion) nor ongoing complaints (vomiting, headache, amnesia, sleepiness, or irritability) are associated with ICI [4,6,8]. In the study by Dietrich and colleagues [6], LOC, amnesia for the event, a GCS of less than 15, and the presence of neurologic deficit were significantly more common in children with ICI. Nevertheless, no single characteristic consistently identified children with ICI because 5% of the neurologically intact patients on presentation had CT scan results that were positive for intracranial pathology.

Glasgow coma scores

GCS scores of 13 to 15 have been considered reflective of MHI, yet patients with ICI can present with these minor scores. In one study among children with GCS 13, 14, or 15, the incidence of intracranial pathology was 33%, 11%, and 5%, respectively [1].

GCS scores can vary depending on the health care professional making the assessment and whether the pediatric GCS system is used. Many times, the adult GCS score is used to evaluate an infant when the pediatric GCS should be used. Hahn and McLone [28] discuss the fact that verbal responses to the GCS system cannot be applied to children under 3 years old. They recommend using the Children's Coma Scale (CCS), which modifies the best verbal response portion of the GCS using the same scale of 3 to 15. Such a scale takes into consideration the different responses that can be expected in a preverbal child (for a more detailed discussion of the Children's Coma Scale, see Hahn, 1993 [28]). Using this scale, pediatric patient responses can be compared with adult responses [28]. In a recent study of pediatric head trauma in children under 2 years of age, the pediatric GCS performed significantly better than the standard GCS applied to older children [30].

The application of the GCS has had mixed results. Wang and colleagues [31] have observed that the distribution of GCS scores did not differ substantially between children who accidentally fell from high- versus low-level heights. Confounding this observation is the finding that 60% of pediatric patients with intracranial hemorrhages were more likely to have improved scores than deteriorated scores in their GCS [25]. However, despite the inconsistency with minor head injury, more severe injuries do correlate with lower coma scores. In a study of head-injured children who required neurosurgical procedures, almost 70% had a GCS less than or equal to 8 [11]. Unfortunately, a normal coma score does not preclude ICI because as many as 28% of patients with ICI are neurologically intact [6]. Ultimately, significant injuries may still exist despite a normal neurologic examination, GCS 13 to 15, or no documented LOC.

Loss of consciousness

Because LOC is believed to be a reliable predictor of ICI, physicians frequently use a history of LOC as an indication to perform CT for the evaluation of head trauma [22,32,33]. Many studies have demonstrated that LOC is a significant indicator of TBI after blunt head injury [3,6,27]. Palchak and colleagues [1] found the risk of TBI to be higher in pediatric patients with a history of LOC or amnesia [34]. In one study of SFs in infants, lethargy (or altered level of consciousness) was the single sign and symptom that was the best positive predictor of ICI (78%) [9].

Conversely, several studies have observed that neither the absence nor the presence of LOC is a significant predictor of negative CT findings [10,24,35]. In the Gruskin and Schutzman study [10], a significant association was found between a depressed level of consciousness and SF or ICI. However, over 90% of the children with isolated SF and 75% of children with ICI (with and without SF) had normal levels of consciousness and nonfocal neurologic examination findings.

Scalp abnormalities

The incidence of SF in children with MHI ranges from 29% to almost 49% [28,35]. Many physicians use the presence of scalp abnormality to dictate ordering radiographic studies. Studies have identified abnormal scalp examinations and SF as important predictors of underlying ICI [1,8,10,24]. The physical finding of a scalp abnormality has been found to have high sensitivity (94%) and negative predictive value (97%) for SF and ICI, and the absence of scalp findings reduces the risk of SF and ICI [10]. In a retrospective study of 401 children with or without brief LOC, a deep scalp wound was the only clinical finding that correlated significantly with positive CT scan findings [35].

   In one study by Greenes and Schutzman [36], scalp hematoma size and location and patient age were useful indicators of SF and underlying ICI in asymptomatic head-injured infants (0–24 months old). Patients with a large or moderate scalp hematoma were significantly more likely to have SFs than patients without scalp hematomas. Parietal and temporal hematomas were both highly associated with SF, and patients with occipital hematomas had a somewhat increased risk for fracture. Younger infants, especially less than 3 months old, had a higher propensity for SF even in the absence of scalp hematoma. A multivariate analysis determined that only a hematoma in the parietal area served as an independent clinical predictor of SF and of ICI. The authors used their data to formulate a scoring system to assess for the risk of SF based on hematoma size and location and patient age. Higher scores, therefore, and a higher risk of SF were assigned to parietal hematoma, large hematoma, and an age less than 3 months. Their decision rule had a sensitivity of 98% and specificity of 49% for detecting SF [36].

   However, SFs do not have to be present for there to be an underlying head injury [7,25,27,37]. Quayle and colleagues [27] have found that the relative risk of ICI increased almost fourfold in the presence of a SF; however, the absence of a SF does not rule out ICI because almost 50% of children with ICI did not have fractures. Similarly, minor craniofacial soft tissue injury (hematoma or laceration) is a significant risk factor for ICI, but it has marginal predictive values [37].

Clinical indicators and management in children less than 2 years old

   The evaluation of the pediatric patient also depends on the age of the patient. Historically, children less than 2 years old have been studied and clinically categorized differently than children older than 2 years. The AAP has published guidelines on the management of minor closed head injury (CHI) in children 2 to 20 years old, but children less than 2 years were not included [33]. Previous authors have excluded children less than 2 years old from their study protocols, which may dampen the portion of children identified with ICI. Children in their first 2 years of life also have been described as being at higher risk for significant brain injury after blunt head trauma. Therefore, infants traditionally have been evaluated differently than older children after head trauma. For example, Masters and colleagues [38] suggest that the age of less than 2 years itself be considered a moderate risk factor for ICI after head trauma. Some authors emphasize a lower threshold as an indication to order imaging studies of younger children because historical and clinical factors may not be available or present for assessment [6]. Many authors make broad recommendations for evaluating infants because even neurologically intact infants may have ICI [7,8,27].

   Younger age can be a strong criterion for identifying the risk of ICI. High incidences of SF and ICI have been found in studies of head-injured children less than 2 years old [6,10,39], with a range from as low as 3.4% [10] to as high to 30% [39]. A multidisciplinary expert panel [32] has defined the factors considered to be higher risk for delayed complications: younger age (especially infants 3–6 months old, who can be more difficult to assess and may lose a significant amount of blood into large scalp hematomas), large scalp swelling, fractures resulting from a high-energy mechanism, and threatening fracture locations (crossing a suture or dural venous sinus, vascular groove, or extending into the posterior fossa) [32].

Some studies have found clinical signs and symptoms to be poor indicators of ICI in infants, and occult ICIs are more common among younger infants [6,33,40]. In the Greenes and Schutzman [40] study of occult ICI in infants less than 2 years old, children were considered symptomatic if they had LOC, a history of behavior change, seizures, vomiting, bulging fontanel, retinal hemorrhages, abnormal neurologic examination, depressed mental status, or irritability. Of the 101 infants studied, 19% had occult ICI. All occult ICIs occurred in infants younger than 1 year, and 95% of the occult ICIs also had SFs.

Although clinical signs and symptoms may be good indicators of either SF or ICI, they are insensitive predictors of head injury in children less than 2 years of age. The combination of the following variables was found in one study to be predictive of SF/ICI: age younger than 12 months, height of fall greater than 3 feet (0.9 m), and scalp abnormality [10]. However, among the subset of children who had fallen and undergone a nonfocal neurologic examination, this combination of variables would identify only 66% of children younger than 2 years with SF/ICI and 72% of children younger than 12 months. Sixty percent of children with SF/ICI had no history of LOC, emesis, seizure, or behavioral change. Furthermore, more than 90% of children with isolated SF and 75% of those with ICI (with or without SF) had nonfocal neurologic examination findings. Therefore, physicians should have a high suspicion for SF/ICI in any child 2 years or younger who has sustained head injury, especially in children younger than 12 months in whom complications are more common and clinical findings are less reliable [10].

Schutzman and colleagues [32] have devised a management strategy that categorizes children less than 2 years old into four subgroups based on the risk of ICI (Box 1). The first group consists of those at high risk for ICI, in whom CT is indicated. The second group consists of those at some risk for ICI, with potential indicators of brain injury in whom CT or observation is indicated. The third group consists of those without potential indicators of brain injury who are at some risk for SF or ICI, in whom CT, skull radiographs, observation is indicated. The fourth group consists of those at low risk for ICI, for whom imaging is not necessary. Generally, the authors emphasize that the younger the patient, the lower the threshold for imaging. The greater the severity and number of historical symptoms and physical signs, the stronger the consideration should be for obtaining an imaging study. Physicians most importantly need to individualize care based on the patient and the unique clinical situation [32].

In conclusion, many authors agree that the greater the forces involved (MVCs, falls from greater heights or onto harder surfaces) and the more pronounced the

Box 1. Management strategy for children less than 2 years old based on the risk of ICI

High risk for ICI: CT scan is recommended

1. Depressed mental status
2. Focal neurologic findings
3. Signs of depressed or basilar SF
4. Acute SF by clinical examination or by skull radiographs
5. Irritability (not easily consoled)
6. Bulging fontanel
7. Seizure[a]
8. Vomiting ≥ 5 times or ≥ 6 per hour[a]
9. *LOC ≥ 1 minute[a]*

Intermediate risk with any potential indicators of brain injury: recommend CT or observation

1. Vomiting, 3 to 4 episodes
2. Transient LOC ≤ 1 minute
3. History of lethargy or irritability, now resolved
4. Behavior not at baseline, reported by caretaker
5. Nonacute SF (≥ 24 hours old)

Intermediate risk with concerning or unknown mechanism or findings on clinical examination that may indicate underlying SF: recommend an imaging procedure (CT, skull radiography, or both) or observation

1. Higher force mechanism (high speed motor vehicle crash or ejection, falls ≥ 3 feet)
2. Falls onto hard surfaces
3. Scalp hematoma (especially if large, boggy, or located in temporoparietal area)
4. Unwitnessed trauma
5. Vague or absent history of trauma in the setting of signs or symptoms of head trauma (should raise the suspicion of child abuse or neglect)

Low risk for ICI: recommend observation

1. Low-energy mechanisms (fall ≤ 3 feet)
2. No signs or symptoms more than 2 hours since injury
3. Older age is more reassuring (especially age ≥ 12 months)

[a] Represents expert consensus.
Adapted from Schutzman et al. Evaluation and management of children younger than two years old with apparently minor head trauma: proposed guidelines. Pediatrics 2001;107:983–93.

physical findings, the greater the risk of ICI. Younger children have a higher incidence of complications, asymptomatic ICI and are more difficult to assess.

Imaging

Skull radiography

Physicians continue to debate the use of skull radiographs to detect underlying head injury. Traditionally, skull radiographs were used to detect a fracture in a child with physical signs of a SF (eg, scalp hematoma). If a fracture was detected by radiography, the follow-up was to perform a head CT. Unfortunately, skull radiographs do not detect underlying brain injury. On the other hand, SFs have been found to be sensitive indicators of ICI in infants [8,27,32,41]. In fact, the presence of a SF is one of the strongest predictors of ICI in children less than 2 years old [32]. The benefits of skull radiographs are that they are readily available and do not require procedural sedation. The value of skull radiographs depends on the accuracy of interpretation because false-positives can stem from open sutures or vascular grooves that appear similar to fractures and vice-versa [41]. Critics of using skull radiography as a screening technique argue that misreading films can incorrectly classify a child as low risk because the fracture has not been identified [41]. Conversely, a child may unnecessarily undergo a head CT when the radiograph incorrectly identifies a fracture.

Studies of pediatric head injury have found that almost half of the ICI occur without a SF present on radiography [25,27]. Additional studies on the ability of plain radiographs to predict ICI have shown a sensitivity of 65% and a negative predictive value of 83%. With a high failure rate of detecting a SF on radiography, there is a large risk of missing a serious brain injury [7]. This high failure rate and poor prediction of underlying ICI have led many investigators to recommend not obtaining skull radiographs when CT is available. However, if CT is not available, skull radiographs can provide screening information, and authors do recommend radiographs in infants younger than 1 year with scalp hematomas or contusions because these infants are at greater risk of SF [27].

CT imaging

To avoid imaging every patient, physicians must decide which child is at risk for ICI and who would benefit from a head CT. The guidelines are clear for children with abnormal examination findings, altered mental status, or major mechanisms of injury. However, the guidelines are less clear for children who present with normal neurologic and physical examination results. Some authors have suggested specific clinical criteria that are indicative of ICI, and these children should have a CT scan [1,2,7,9,27], yet other authors have found clinical criteria to be inadequate as screening tests for ICI [4,6,8,35]. Articles have discussed the use of CT scan of children after MHI, which would conceivably identify all potentially life-threatening ICI. However, there is likely a subgroup of children in whom the potential for ICI is so low that the benefits of CT scans do not justify the costs [24].

The indications for CT scanning in minor pediatric head trauma remain controversial. Guidelines for imaging a child with a minor injury are ill defined and subjective to the practitioner and institution. One author points out that a liberal policy of CT scanning should be adopted in pediatric patients with significant mechanisms of injury despite normal findings on neurologic examination. Early CT scanning would capture the few patients who may require neurosurgical intervention [37]. In addition, CT scanning should be considered in any neurologically intact child who shows significant signs of brain injury (LOC, amnesia for the event, vomiting, seizures, headache, and focal neurologic deficits) [6].

With the increasing availability of CT, physicians face the conflict of selecting the patients who would benefit from obtaining the scan, yet they are confronted with the consequences of failing to diagnose ICI if scanning is not done. The use of CT scan as a method of pediatric MHI evaluation must be weighed against health care costs, time-consuming measures for staff, the need for procedural sedation, overall ED visit times, lost parental work time and wages, travel expenses, and parental anxiety [6,42]. A 2000 Canadian study compared the usage rates of CT scans at nine pediatric hospitals [3]. The authors reported a significant difference in the rate of ordering CT scans (6%–26%) among the participating hospitals but no significant difference in the rate of abnormal CT scans (1%–9%). Reasons posited for the various usage rates are the differing criteria for imaging among clinicians, the availability of CT scanning at the various hospitals, and the differences in the patient populations. Nevertheless, the frequencies of positive findings on CT scans did not differ based on the number of scans ordered.

Radiation risk has been a concern for children who undergo CT scanning after head injury [11,43–45]. Unfortunately, higher radiation doses improve image quality, and children receive a higher radiation dose than older children or adults for the same CT settings [46]. Likewise, children have a longer postimaging lifetime in which to manifest radiation-related cancer, and the cancer risk is cumulative over time. The increase in cancer risk has been reported to be as low as 0.35% for overall lifetime risk [43]. Authorities have also suggested that instead of omitting CT scanning, adjusting CT scanners to appropriate setting for the small heads of children might be sufficient to balance the risks and benefits of CT imaging [43,46].

American Academy of Pediatrics mild head injury guidelines

The AAP has published a practice parameter for the management of minor CHI in children [33]. The Committee on Quality Improvement of the AAP worked in collaboration with the Commission on Clinical Policies and Research of the American Academy of Family Physicians and experts in neurology, emergency medicine and critical care, research methodologists, and practicing physicians. The practice parameter makes recommendations for managing previously neurologically healthy children ages 2 to 20 who suffer minor CHIs. On presentation, the child may have experienced a temporary LOC (≤ 1 minute), an impact seizure, vomiting, or other signs and symptoms. The parameter defines children with minor CHI as those who have normal mental status at the initial examination, no abnormal or focal findings on neurologic examination (including fundoscopic), and have no physical evidence of SF. The parameter is not intended for victims of multiple trauma, children who have unobserved LOC, or patients who have known or suspected cervical spine injury. Finally, the parameter is directed only to the management of children evaluated by a health care professional within 24 hours after the injury.

For children with CHI and no LOC, a thorough history and an appropriate physical and neurologic examination should be performed, followed by observation. Observation includes the setting of the clinic, office, ED or at home, under the care of a competent caregiver. The use of CT, skull radiography, or MRI is not recommended. If the patient's findings on examination appear normal, no additional tests are needed, and the child may be discharged under the care of a responsible guardian. The Quality Standards Subcommittee of the AAN [16] believes that the low prevalence of ICI and the marginal benefits of early detection of ICI afforded by imaging studies were outweighed by the considerations of cost, resource allocation, inconvenience, and possible side effects of sedation. The parameter discusses the limited role of skull radiographs in evaluating children with MHI, no LOC, and no signs of SF. Some situations may arise in which the physician may order an imaging study (eg, scalp hematoma over the course of meningeal artery). The Subcommittee believes that cranial CT scanning is the imaging modality of choice based on its increased sensitivity and specificity and the low predictive value of skull radiographs. When CT is not available, skull radiography may assist the practitioner in determining the risk for ICI. For children with minor CHI and brief LOC (≤ 1 minute), the parameter recommends observation or cranial CT scan. However, skull radiography and MRI are not recommended.

Disposition

Multiple factors contribute to the decision on whether to admit a child after head trauma. Some of these factors involve concerns of associated injuries, neurologic observation, and the child's home environment. Many children who sustain isolated MHI have traditionally been hospitalized for observation, despite normal findings on neurologic examination and even on imaging studies. Most of these patients do well and do not have adverse events during their admission [28,35,47–49].

Several prospective studies have shown that normal CT scans and normal examinations may be helpful criteria in deciding to safely discharge patients from the ED. In three studies (a total of 261 patients), there was a late deterioration incidence rate of zero in children with normal CT results [4,8,22,27]. Similarly, in six studies (a total of 349 patients) there was a zero incidence rate for clinical deterioration for children with isolated SF and no ICI present [4,8,9,22,27,50,51]. Several other trials demonstrate that in otherwise stable patients with a normal mental status, cranial CT and neurologic examination can be performed and the patient can be safely discharged from the ED [24,42,47]. A thorough evaluation, including normal physical examination and neuroimaging, would be more cost-effective than 1 to 2 days of hospital observation [42]. A large study that provided a comprehensive statewide follow-up of 400 children who had normal CT scan results after head injury observed that the children remained stable after discharge [42]. Only four children had delayed symptoms requiring hospitalization, and only one required operative neurosurgical management (this patient had a known risk factor for a bleeding diathesis). Many authors have demonstrated that patients with a normal CT scan and neurologic assessment after MHI are at very low risk for subsequent intracranial bleeding or neurologic sequelae and may be discharged from the ED if a competent observer is available [42,47,49].

Outcome and seizures

The short- and long-term complications of MHI in children are poorly understood. Studies have investigated both short-term and long-term outcome from MHI, specifically studying symptoms and behavioral and cognitive effects. The term postconcussive syndrome refers to the constellation of acute symptoms after MHI. These symptoms can be somatic (headache, dizziness, blurriness), emotional (irritability, anxiety), and cognitive (concentration and memory) [18]. The complete diagnostic criteria for postconcussive syndrome can be found in the "International Statistical Classification of Diseases and Related Health Problems," 10th edition [52].

Short-term outcome

Hahn and McLone [28] studied the risk factors in the outcome of children who had MHI. In their prospective study of admitted children, 84% had minor head injuries. Of the 780 children who lost consciousness for 0 to 15 minutes, none had a poor outcome (defined as suffering severe disabilities, vegetative state, or death). Almost 6% developed various forms of seizures after the trauma. The authors did not find a statistical difference between CCS scores and the incidence of posttraumatic seizure. However, children with seizures had twice the risk of having a poor outcome ($P = .001$). Of the 94% who did not have seizures, 3% had a poor outcome, compared with 6.4% of the children who had seizures with a poor outcome. The authors found that children with punctate hemorrhages on CT scans did not have an additional risk of a poorer outcome than children did with normal CT scans ($P = .001$).

Studies have assessed physical, behavioral, and cognitive outcomes across the severity continuum of head injuries. Pavlovitch and colleagues [53] determined that speech and feeding difficulties were associated with an increasing severity of head injury, whereas walking was not. Headaches are among the most common postconcussive symptoms reported, but most headaches are resolved several months after injury [27,54–56]. Similarly, temper outbursts, dizziness, mood swings, anxiety, and aggressive behavior have been reported more significantly across the injury severity continuum. In one study, the parents of 28% of the children believed that the personality of their child had changed since the head injury, with significantly more reporting the higher the severity of head injury [54]. Another study of children with MHI reported more symptoms than controls at 1 week but did not demonstrate impairment on neuropsychologic measures [56]. Initial symptoms had resolved for most children by 3 months after the injury, but there was a group of children (17%) whose parents continued to report symptoms and behavioral problems. These children who had ongoing problems were more likely to have had a previous head injury, neurologic or psychiatric problems, a history of learning or behavioral difficulties, or family stressors. The authors emphasize that the "at risk" children who have the potential for poorer outcomes should be identified in the emergency department and monitored through follow-up. A similar study by the same authors, found that a careful assessment and providing an information booklet and coping strategies resulted in significantly reduced anxiety as well as reports of symptoms and behavioral changes 3 months after injury [55].

Children with MHI do well in their recovery, but studies have found that not all mildly injured children recover completely. In the study by Hawley and colleagues [54], half of the study group made a good recovery, but only 18.4% made a full recovery without discernible sequelae. The most frequent reason for placing a child in the good but not full recovery category was the presence of headaches. The authors state that a surprising number of children with MHI had moderate disability (43%) at follow-up. The authors were unable to identify a threshold of injury severity below which the risk of late morbidity could be discounted.

Long-term outcome

The long-term outcome after MHI continues to be a controversy. Satz and colleagues [57] performed a review of 40 outcome studies between 1970 and

1995, specifically examining three outcomes: neuropsychologic, academic, and psychosocial. Of the 40 studies, the results of the comprehensive review revealed 13 adverse, 18 null, and 9 indeterminate findings related to the three outcomes of interest. They did not find adverse effects on academic or psychosocial outcomes across the spectrum of MHI or on neuropsychologic outcomes at the more extreme end of the MHI distribution. When the studies were classified based on methodological merit, the stronger studies were generally associated with null outcomes. The authors concluded that MHI in children may result in mild but transitory alteration in cognitive functioning (attention and memory) but no reliable changes in academic or psychologic functioning. However, because severity within the MHI spectrum increased, more variability in findings was reported, and there may be a degree of mild injury that reaches a threshold of concern.

Authors have studied extensively the effects of MHI on measures of behavior, cognition, and physical and family functioning. Children with MHI recover fairly well, and those who experience more severe head injury are more likely to have long-term negative outcomes. Anderson and colleagues [58] examined the effect of MHI in young children (3–7 years old) using standardized measures of adaptive, behavioral, and cognitive functioning at the time of initial hospitalization and at 6 and 30 months after injury. No significant differences were noted between the study group and the matched controls on most cognitive measures (intellectual, speed of processing, attention, memory, receptive vocabulary, and auditory comprehension), both at the acute stage and at 30 months after injury. The MHI group performed significantly worse than the control group did on story recall and verbal fluency, suggesting that MHI may produce impairment in certain high-level language skills. The MHI group improved over time, and the authors comment that these impairments were transient interruptions of brain functions and delay in skill acquisition rather than permanent deficits. The authors conclude that children with MHI have generally good outcomes during the preschool years [59]. In another study by Anderson and colleagues [59], it was observed that a dose-response relationship exists for injury severity and physical and cognitive outcomes. Behavioral functioning was not related to injury severity, although results approached significance. For physical and cognitive recovery (acutely after injury and at 30 months), injury severity was a consistent predictor along with socioeconomic status. After injury, the child and family function were less associated with injury factors and more dependent on preinjury psychosocial functions. The authors conclude that preinjury factors play a key role in postinjury behavior and family function, which suggests that premorbid vulnerabilities increase the risk of poor outcome after TBI.

Another study examined long-term psychosocial outcomes after MHI in early childhood [60]. This study showed that children who experienced a MHI of sufficient severity to warrant temporary hospitalization between ages of 0 to 10 years old were likely to show adverse psychosocial outcomes in terms of hyperactivity and inattention and conduct-disordered behavior at 10 to 13 years of age, especially if the injury occurred before the age of 5. In contrast, children in the outpatient MHI group were comparable to the noninjured reference group on psychosocial measures. The authors concluded that long-term psychosocial problems may be more likely at the upper end of the MHI severity spectrum.

When children with head injury return to school, they may be expected to assimilate immediately with the class. The child's teacher may not understand the head injury or even know the child suffered a MHI, which could affect how the child is treated, observed, or graded. In the study by Hawley and colleagues [54], teachers knew of the child's head injury in only 39.8% of the children, and there was a significant linear trend across injury severity groups. Special educational needs were provided for only 65% of the children identified with such needs, which did show a significant linear trend across injury severity. At follow-up, 18.7% of the children were currently having difficulties with schoolwork, and there was a significant linear trend across severity groups. Interestingly, 18% of the children had been disciplined by the school for problem behavior after sustaining their head injury [54].

Posttraumatic seizure

Posttraumatic seizures (PTS) after MHI can be relatively common in children. Recent studies cite a 3% to 6% incidence of PTS [28,61]. Rarely do these children need treatment, but children with PTS traditionally have been admitted to the hospital for observation. PTS can be defined as immediate (occurring within 24 hours of the head injury), early (occurring between 24 hours and 7 days after the injury), and late (occurring beyond 7 days after the injury) [62]. Impact seizures have also been described as developing at the time of the accident [28].

PTS after blunt head trauma may be associated with the presence of TBI. Although some studies indicate that mildly injured children without PTS who have normal findings on neurologic examinations and head CT scans do not need routine hospitalization, some authors have questioned the traditional admission of children after PTS [61,62]. Studies have found that hospitalized patients after both MHI and PTS do well without any further seizure activity and normal neurologic exams. These authors emphasize that children who have isolated head injury and simple PTS who recover fully in the ED, whose CT scans do not show any ICI and no history of neurologic disease, are at low risk for recurrent seizures or neurologic complications. The authors suggest that these low-risk patients can potentially be sent home with a reliable caregiver [61,62].

The discussion of which child with PTS requires admission and which child can be discharged from the ED focuses on the question of what is the risk of sending home a child who suffered an uncomplicated PTS. Studies have found that the risk of PTS is more frequent among patients who have abnormal head CT scan results and altered mental status and that these patients are at higher risk for requiring neurosurgical procedures [61,63]. If all children with PTS have cranial CT scans, then a normal scan helps to eliminate that risk. Another concern is the risk of a prolonged seizure or status epilepticus. Furthermore, younger children have inconsistently been found to be more likely to suffer PTS. In the study by Dias and colleagues [62], children with immediate PTS were significantly younger than a control group of children with uncomplicated MHI, 11% of the children had a prolonged seizure (≥ 5 min) and were treated with anticonvulsants and admitted to the ICU. Sixty-five percent of the children had the first seizure within 1 hour of impact, and 72% of the children studied had only a single seizure, yet no child suffered additional seizures or significant complications. The authors therefore concluded that as many as 85% of these children could have been discharged to home after normal imaging studies and a return to normal function after a single or brief seizure.

Seizure prophylaxis has been studied mostly in patients with moderate to severe head injuries. A 2004 randomized controlled trial studied phenytoin versus placebo in 102 patients 16 years old or less [64]. These children had a more serious head injury because the requirement for enrollment was GCS of 9 or 10, depending on age. The study did not find a significant difference in the rate of early PTS in the phenytoin versus placebo group.

Sports injuries

Recent research and news headlines on head injuries in athletes have raised concerns over the health of athletes who sustain concussions. Furthermore, these discussions have motivated clinicians and sports medicine specialists to develop practice guidelines and parameters for evaluating and managing the head-injured athlete. The various guidelines released have raised controversy because scientific foundation and delineation of concussion grades and return-to-play criteria are lacking [65]. In addition, there has been disagreement over the potential negative outcome of cumulative concussions. So far, there is no consensus on tests that assess baseline and posttraumatic neuropsychologic function. To begin the discussion of managing concussions in sports, physicians and researchers must have a common understanding and definition of what constitutes a concussion.

Many definitions of concussion have been proposed, but there is no universally accepted definition. Often, the term concussion has been used interchangeably with MHI [20]. The AAN defines concussion as "a trauma-induced alteration in mental status that may or may not involve loss of consciousness" and states that confusion and amnesia are hallmarks of concussion [16]. Many of the classifications of MHI and guidelines for management have been generated from studies of athletic injuries [20]. An agreement on a precise definition of concussion and the subtle delineations would help to solidify the general cohesiveness of how practitioners evaluate and manage athletes with concussions.

The three popular grading scales and guidelines are those of Cantu, the Sports Medicine Committee of the Colorado Medical Society, and the AAN (Table 1). In 1988, Cantu [66] developed guidelines for concussion by modifying the definition set earlier by the Congress of Neurological Surgeons and incorporated posttraumatic amnesia (PTA) into the definition. Cantu graded sports-related

Table 1
Concussion grading schemes

Cantu	American Academy of Neurology	Colorado Medical Society
Grade 1 (mild)	Grade 1	Grade 1
No LOC	No LOC	No LOC
PTA ≤30 min	Transient confusion	Transient confusion
	Symptoms resolve ≤15 min	No PTA
Grade 2 (moderate)	Grade 2	Grade 2
LOC ≤5 min, or	No LOC	No LOC
PTA ≥30 min	Transient confusion	Confusion with PTA
	Symptoms last ≥15 min	
Grade 3 (severe)	Grade 3	Grade 3
LOC ≥5 min, or	Any LOC, brief or prolonged	LOC of any duration
PTA ≥24 h		

Data from Refs. [16,65,67].

concussions on the length of unconsciousness and PTA. In 1991, Kelly and colleagues worked with the Sports Medicine Committee of the Colorado Medical Society to develop another definition with associated guidelines [67,68]. Each level of concussion (mild, moderate, and severe) was described according to the length of unconsciousness and confusion or amnesia. The misunderstanding that concussion requires LOC still exists, and thus Kelly and colleagues reiterate that concussion should be defined as a traumatically induced alteration in mental status [67]. In 1997, the Quality Standards Subcommittee of the AAN developed a concussion severity rating scale in which both confusion and amnesia are important characteristics of concussion designations [16].

In 2001 and 2004, a panel of experts [69] met for an international symposium on concussion in sports and revised a consensus definition of sports concussion originally developed by the Committee on Head Injury Nomenclature of the Congress of Neurological Surgeons. The updated definition describes a sports concussion "as a complex pathophysiologic process affecting the brain, induced by traumatic biomechanical forces" [69]. Further delineations are made about concussion, stating that it is typically of rapid onset and a short-lived impairment of neurologic function that resolves spontaneously. In addition, concussion is typically associated with grossly normal structural neuroimaging studies. The group [69] proposed a new classification of concussion in sports as either simple or complex. In a simple concussion, an athlete suffers an injury that progressively resolves without complication over 7 to 10 days. Formal neuropsychologic screening does not play a role in these circumstances, although mental status screening should be a part of the assessment. The cornerstone of management is rest until all symptoms resolve. The group emphasized that all concussions mandate evaluation by a medical doctor; however, a simple concussion can be managed by a primary care physician or certified athletic trainer who has medical supervision. On the other hand, in a complex concussion, an athlete suffers persistent symptoms, specific sequelae (eg, prolonged LOC over 1 min), or prolonged cognitive impairment after the injury. This classification may also include athletes who

Table 2
Return-to-play guidelines for concussion grading scales

System	Grade 1	Grade 2	Grade 3
Cantu [66] 1988	Athlete may return to play that day in select situations if normal clinical examination at rest and exertion; if symptomatic, athlete may return to play in 7 days	Athlete may return to play in 2 wk if asymptomatic at rest and exertion for 7 d	Athlete may return to play in 1 mo if asymptomatic at rest and exertion for 7 d
Colorado Medical Society [68] 1991	Remove athlete from contest and examine immediately and every 5 min; permit return to contest if amnesia or symptoms do not appear for 20 min	Remove from contest and disallow return; examine athlete next day; permit return to practice after 1 wk without symptoms	Transport athlete to hospital and perform neurologic exam; admit to hospital if signs of pathology are detected, otherwise overnight observation; permit return to practice if asymptomatic for 2 wk
American Academy of Neurology [16] 1997	Examine athlete immediately for mental status changes; may return to contest if no symptoms or mental status changes at 15 min	Remove athlete from contest and disallow return; examine athlete on site for symptoms or mental status changes; athlete may return in 1 wk if asymptomatic	Remove athlete from contest and transport to hospital; perform neurologic exam and observe overnight; permit return to play if asymptomatic after 1 wk (if LOC was brief) or 2 wk (if LOC was prolonged)

Data from Refs. [16,65–68].

suffer multiple concussions over time. Athletes with complex concussions should be managed by physicians with specific expertise in the management of concussive injury [69].

The management and return-to-play guidelines also differ among Cantu, the Colorado Medical Society, and the AAN (Table 2). The Colorado system distinguishes between grade 1 and 2 concussions according to the presence of symptoms, whereas the AAN makes this distinction according to the duration of symptoms [70]. Depending on which guideline is followed, an athlete may return to play at drastically different times, which may be too conservative or too hasty [65].

Second impact syndrome

The term "second impact syndrome" was first coined by Saunders and Harbaugh in 1984 [71]. Cantu has defined second impact syndrome as an injury in which "an athlete who has sustained an initial head injury, most often a concussion, sustains a second head injury before symptoms associated with the first have fully cleared" [72]. The syndrome can propel a rapid cascade of cerebral vascular congestion, causing increased intracranial pressure and brainstem herniation and ultimately may lead to death [73]. McCrory and colleagues established criteria for definite, probable, and possible second impact syndrome and did not find any definite cases of second impact syndrome [74].

Many reports of complications and even death have been attributed to second impact syndrome; however, the diagnosis remains controversial. Maroon and colleagues [20] state that second impact syndrome "is an infrequent finding, predominately involves young athletes, and only rarely is fatal." To prevent the second impact syndrome, popular guidelines have recommended that athletes not return to play until the postconcussive symptoms have resolved [16,67,68]. The delayed development of amnesia or postconcussive symptoms suggests that some pathologic processes occur gradually and could be missed if an athlete returns to play too early [67]. Kelly and colleagues [75] emphasize that prematurely returning to sports in which head injury is a risk could lead to a catastrophic outcome such as permanent disability or death.

Neuropsychologic testing of athletes

Most of the neuropsychologic testing of patients has been on adults or professional or amateur athletes of near adult age. Neuropsychologic testing for patients after mild TBI involves systematically testing the athlete at the beginning of the season for a baseline comparison, then 24 hours after the head injury, and then again at 5 days. Baseline assessments are essential to the neuropsychologic test because any deficits in the athlete's performance need to be detected and attributed to the effects of the concussion or to previous unrelated factors [20].

Several studies have examined recovery from mild concussion in high school athletes. Researches have tried to identify diagnostic markers of concussion severity and how the markers relate to recovery. In a study of high school athletes who suffered mild concussion, the authors found significant declines in memory processes relative to the noninjured control group. Statistically significant differences between preseason and postinjury memory test results were still evident in the concussion group at 4 and 7 days after the injury. Self-reported neurologic symptoms, such as headache, dizziness, and nausea had resolved by day 4. The authors observed that on-field mental status changes such as retrograde amnesia and confusion were related to the presence of memory impairment at 36 hours and 4 and 7 days after injury as was also related to slower resolution of self-reported symptoms. The authors conclude that on-field mental status changes appear to have prognostic value and should be taken into account when making return-to-play decisions [76].

Chronic traumatic brain injury (CTBI) is the cumulative long-term neurologic consequence of repetitive and subconcussive blows to the head. Matser and colleagues [77] studied 33 amateur soccer players and 27 controls (amateur swimmers and runners) to determine whether soccer players had evidence of CTBI. Compared with the control athletes, the amateur soccer players exhibited impaired performance on tests of planning and memory. The authors found that the number of concussions incurred in soccer was inversely related to the neuro-psychologic performance on six of 16 tests. The authors conclude that the findings suggest participation in amateur soccer may be associated with CTBI, as evidenced by impairment on cognitive functioning [77].

Researches have tried to answer the question, how many concussions are too many? Collins and colleagues [78] assessed the relationship between concussion history and learning disability and the association of these variables with neuro-psychologic performance. Of 393 college football players with a mean age of 20.4 years, 34% had experienced one previous concussion and 20% had experienced two or more concussions. The authors observed that both a history of multiple concussions and learning disability were associated with reduced cognitive performance. A history of concussion was significantly associated with deficits in domains of executive functioning and the speed of information processing. The authors found that a history of one concussion does not result in the long-term cognitive morbidity that is associated with two or more episodes of concussion. As commonly agreed, any neurologic symptom should signal that full recovery was not completed and that return to play was contraindicated. The authors suggest that neuropsychologic testing may detect subtle cognitive impairments and that mental status screening instruments are variable and may miss the subtle deficits associated with head injury [78]. Each concussion needs to be evaluated individually and correlated with appropriate neuropsychologic tests as well as neuroimaging studies [20].

Summary

Many studies have found conflicting evidence over the use of clinical indicators to predict ICI in pediatric MHI. Although altered mental status, LOC, and abnormal neurologic examination findings have all been found to be more prevalent among head-injured children, studies have observed inconsistent results over their specificity and predictive value. Children older than 2 years have been evaluated, managed, and studied differently than those younger than 2 years. Evidence strongly supports a lower threshold for performing a CT scan in younger children because they have a higher risk of significant brain injury after blunt head trauma.

Many authors state that children with MHI who have normal CT scan results and normal mental status and neurologic examination findings may be discharged from the ED with a reliable caregiver and detailed head injury instructions. Further research involving multicenter trials with prospective enrollment will help to validate the decision making and previous recommendations on neuroimaging, hospitalization, observation, and discharge. Currently, the Pediatric Emergency Care Applied Research Network is conducting a multicenter study to address these questions. This study is currently in progress and has enrolled 16,000 children, with plans to enroll over 25,000 children. One of the goals is to create a neuroimaging decision rule on children with minor to moderate head trauma.

Most children with MHI make a full recovery; however, a subset of children with preinjury morbidity may develop neuropsychologic sequelae. The management of sports-related head injuries demands identifying potential neurosurgical emergencies and preventing catastrophic outcomes related to acute brain swelling and repetitive concussions.

References

[1] Palchak MJ, Holmes JF, Vance CW, et al. A decision rule for identifying children at low risk for brain injuries after blunt head trauma. Ann Emerg Med 2003;42(4):492–506.

[2] Haydel MJ, Shembekar AD. Prediction of intracranial injury in children aged five years and older with loss of consciousness after minor head injury due to nontrivial mechanisms. Ann Emerg Med 2003;42(4):507–14.

[3] Klassen TP, Reed MH, Stiell IG, et al. Variation in utilization of computed tomography scanning for the investigation of minor head trauma in children: a Canadian experience. Acad Emerg Med 2000;7(7):739–44.

[4] Schunk JE, Rodgerson JD, Woodward GA. The utility of head computed tomographic scanning in pediatric patients with normal neurologic examination in the emergency department. Pediatr Emerg Care 1996;12(3):160–5.

[5] Bazarian JJ, McClung J, Shah MN, et al. Mild traumatic brain injury in the United States, 1998–2000. Brain Inj 2005;19(2):85–91.

[6] Dietrich AM, Bowman MJ, Ginn-Pease ME, et al. Pediatric head injuries: can clinical factors reliably predict an abnormality on computed tomography? Ann Emerg Med 1993;22(10):1535–40.

[7] Lloyd DA, Carty H, Patterson M, et al. Predictive value of skull radiography for intracranial injury in children with blunt head injury. Lancet 1997;349:821–4.

[8] Greenes DS, Schutzman SA. Clinical indicators for intracranial injury in head-injured infants. Pediatrics 1999;104(4):861–7.

[9] Shane SA, Fuchs SM. Skull fractures in infants and predictors of associated intracranial injury. Pediatr Emerg Care 1997;13(3):198–203.

[10] Gruskin KD, Schutzman SA. Head trauma in children younger than 2 years: are there predictors for complications? Arch Pediatr Adolesc Med 1999;153:15–20.

[11] Brown L, Moynihan JA, Denmark TK. Blunt pediatric head trauma requiring neurosurgical intervention: how subtle can it be? Am J Emerg Med 2003;21(6):467–72.

[12] American Academy of Pediatrics, Committee on Injury and Poison Prevention. Injury associated with infant walkers. Pediatrics 2001;108(3):790–2.

[13] Shafi S, Gilbert JC, Lodhmanee F, et al. Impact of bicycle helmet safety legislation on children admitted to a regional pediatric trauma center. J Pediatr Surg 1998;33(2):317–21.

[14] MacPherson AK, To TM, Macarthur C, et al. Impact of mandatory helmet legislation on bicycle-related head injuries in children: a population-based study. Pediatrics 2002;110(5):60–5.

[15] Bazarian JJ. Helmets for preventing head, brain, and facial injuries in cyclists. Ann Emerg Med 2003;41(5):738–40.

[16] Quality Standards Subcommittee, American Academy of Neurology. Practice parameter: the management of concussion in sports (summary statement). Neurology 1997;48(3):581–5.

[17] Mild Traumatic Brain Injury Committee of the Head Injury Interdisciplinary Special Interest Group of American Congress of Rehabilitation Medicine. Definition of mild traumatic brain injury. J Head Trauma Rehabil 1993;8:86–7.

[18] Thompson MD, Irby Jr JW. Recovery from mild head injury in pediatric populations. Semin Pediatr Neurol 2003;10(2):130–9.

[19] Savitsky EA, Votey SR. Current controversies in the management of minor pediatric head injuries. Am J Emerg Med 2000;18(1):96–101.

[20] Maroon JC, Lovell MR, Norwig J, et al. Cerebral concussion in athletes: evaluation and neuropsychological testing. Neurosurgery 2000;47(3):659–72.

[21] Ghajar J, Hariri RJ. Management of pediatric head injury. Pediatr Clin North Am 1992;39(5): 1093–125.

[22] Schutzman SA, Greenes DS. Pediatric minor head trauma. Ann Emerg Med 2001;37(1):65–74.

[23] Woestman R, Perkin R, Serna T, et al. Mild head injury in children: identification, clinical evaluation, neuroimaging, and disposition. Int J Trauma Nurs 1999;5(2):49–62.

[24] Davis RL, Mullen N, Makela M, et al. Cranial computed tomography scans in children after minimal head injury with loss of consciousness. Ann Emerg Med 1994;24(4):640–5.

[25] Wang MY, Griffith P, Sterling J, et al. A prospective population-based study of pediatric trauma patients with mild alterations in consciousness (Glasgow Coma Scale Score of 13-14). Neurosurgery 2000;46(5):1093–9.

[26] Ramundo ML, McKnight T, Kempf J, et al. Clinical predictors of computed tomographic abnormalities following pediatric traumatic brain injury. Pediatr Emerg Care 1995;11(1):1–4.

[27] Quayle KS, Jaffe DM, Kuppermann N, et al. Diagnostic testing for acute head injury in children: when are head computed tomography and skull radiographs indicated? Pediatrics 1998;99(5): 1–8.

[28] Hahn YS, McLone DG. Risk factors in the outcome of children with minor head injury. Pediatr Neurosurg 1993;19:135–42.

[29] Halley MK, Silva PD, Foley J, et al. Loss of consciousness: when to perform computed tomography? Pediatr Crit Care Med 2004;5(3):230–3.

[30] Palchak MH, Holmes JF, MacFarlane TI, et al. Performance of the pediatric Glasgow Coma Scale in pediatric head trauma. Acad Emerg Med 2003;10(5):497.

[31] Wang MY, Kim KA, Griffith PM, et al. Injuries from falls in the pediatric population: an analysis of 729 cases. J Pediatr Surg 2001;36(10):1528–34.

[32] Schutzman SA, Barnes P, Duhaime AC, et al. Evaluation and management of children younger than two years old with apparently minor head trauma: proposed guidelines. Pediatrics 2001; 107(5):983–93.

[33] American Academy of Pediatrics. The management of minor closed head injury in children. Pediatrics 1999;104(6):1407–15.

[34] Palchak MJ, Holmes JF, Vance CW, et al. Does an isolated history of loss of consciousness or amnesia predict brain injuries in children after blunt head trauma? Pediatrics 2004;113(6): 507–13.

[35] Mitchell KA, Fallat ME, Raque GH, et al. Evaluation of minor head injury in children. J Pediatr Surg 1994;29(7):851–4.

[36] Greenes DS, Schutzman SA. Clinical significance of scalp abnormalities in asymptomatic head-injured infants. Pediatr Emerg Care 2001;17(2):88–92.

[37] Simon B, Letourneau P, Vitorino E, et al. Pediatric minor head trauma: indications for computed tomography revisited. J Trauma 2001;51(2):231–8.

[38] Masters SJ, McClean PM, Arcarese JS, et al. Skull x-ray examinations after head trauma: recommendations by a multidisciplinary panel and validation study. N Engl J Med 1987;316(2): 84–91.

[39] Duhaime AC, Alario AJ, Lewander WJ, et al. Head injury in very young children: mechanisms, injury types, and ophthalmologic findings in 100 hospitalized patients younger than 2 years of age. Pediatrics 1992;90(2):179–85.

[40] Greenes DS, Schutzman SA. Occult intracranial injury in infants. Ann Emerg Med 1998; 32(6):680–6.

[41] Chung S, Schamban N, Wypij D, et al. Skull radiograph interpretation of children younger than two years: how good are pediatric emergency physicians? Ann Emerg Med 2004;43(6): 718–22.

[42] Davis RL, Hughes M, Gubler KD, et al. The use of cranial CT scans in the triage of pediatric patients with mild head injury. Pediatrics 1995;95(3):345–9.

[43] Brenner DJ, Elliston CD, Hall EJ, et al. Estimated risks of radiation-induced fatal cancer from pediatric CT. Am J Radiol 2001;176:289–96.

[44] Paterson A, Frush FP, Donnelly LF. Helical CT of the body: are settings adjusted for pediatric patients? Am J Radiol 2001;176:297–301.

[45] Donnelly LF, Emery KH, Brody AS, et al. Minimizing radiation dose for pediatric body applications of single-detector helical CT: strategies at a large children's hospital. Am J Radiol 2001;176:303–6.

[46] Frush DP, Donnelly LF, Rosen NS. Computed tomography and radiation risks: what pediatric health care providers should know. Pediatrics 2003;112(4):951–7.

[47] Roddy SP, Cohn SM, Moller BA, et al. Minimal head trauma in children revisited: is routine hospitalization required? Pediatrics 1998;101(4):575–7.

[48] Adams J, Frumiento C, Shatney-Leach L, et al. Mandatory admission after isolated mild closed head injury in children: is it necessary? J Pediatr Surg 2001;36(1):119–21.

[49] Spencer MT, Bonny JB, Sinert R, et al. Necessity of hospital admission for pediatric minor head injury. Am J Emerg Med 2003;21(2):111–4.

[50] Greenes DS, Schutzman SA. Infants with isolated skull fracture: what are their clinical characteristics, and do they require hospitalization? Ann Emerg Med 1997;30(3):253–9.

[51] Partington M, Swanson J, Meyer F. Head injury and the use of baby walkers. Ann Emerg Med 1991;20:652–4.

[52] World Health Organization. International statistical classification of diseases and related health problems. 10th edition. Geneva, Switzerland: World Health Organization; 1992.

[53] Pavlovitch C, DiRusso SM, Risucci D, et al. Mortality and functional outcome in pediatric trauma patients with and without head injuries. Acad Emerg Med 2003;10(5):495–6.

[54] Hawley CA, Ward AB, Magnay AR, et al. Outcomes following head injury: a population study. J Neurol Neurosurg Psychiatry 2004;75:737–42.

[55] Ponsford J, Willmott C, Rothwell A, et al. Impact of early intervention on outcome after mild traumatic brain injury in children. Pediatrics 2001;108(6):1297–303.

[56] Ponsford J, Willmott C, Rothwell A, et al. Cognitive and behavioral outcome following mild traumatic head injury in children. J Head Trauma Rehabil 1999;14(4):360–72.

[57] Satz P, Zaucha K, Light R, et al. Mild head injury in children and adolescents: a review of studies (1970–1995). Psychol Bull 1997;122(2):107–31.

[58] Anderson VA, Catroppa C, Morse S, et al. Outcome from mild head injury in young children: a prospective study. J Clin Exp Neuropsychol 2001;23:705–17.

[59] Anderson VA, Catroppa C, Haritou F, et al. Identifying factors contributing to child and family outcome 30 months after traumatic brain injury in children. J Neurol Neurosurg Psychiatry 2005;76:401–8.

[60] McKinlay A, Dairymple-Alford JC, Horwood LJ, et al. Long term psychosocial outcomes after mild head injury in early childhood. J Neurol Neurosurg Psychiatry 2002;73:281–8.

[61] Holmes JF, Palchak MJ, Conklin MJ, et al. Do children require hospitalization after immediate posttraumatic seizures? Ann Emerg Med 2004;43(6):706–10.

[62] Dias MS, Carnevale F, Li V. Immediate posttraumatic seizures: is routine hospitalization necessary? Pediatr Neurosurg 1999;30:232–8.

[63] Lewis RJ, Yee L, Inkelis SH, et al. Clinical predictors of posttraumatic seizures in children with head trauma. Ann Emerg Med 1993;22:1114–8.

[64] Young KD, Okada PJ, Sokolove PE, et al. A randomized double-blinded placebo-controlled trial of phenytoin for the prevention of early posttraumatic seizures in children with moderate to severe blunt head injury. Ann Emerg Med 2004;43(4):435–46.

[65] Collins MW, Lovell MR, McKeag DB. Current issues in managing sports-related concussion. JAMA 1999;282(24):2283–5.

[66] Cantu RC. When to return to contact sports after a cerebral concussion. Sports Med Digest 1988; 10:1–2.

[67] Kelly JP, Nichols JS, Filley CM, et al. Concussion in sports: guidelines for the prevention of catastrophic outcome. JAMA 1991;266(20):2867–9.

[68] Colorado Medical Society. Report of the sports medicine committee: guidelines for the management of concussions in sport (revised). Denver: Colorado Medical Society; 1991.

[69] McCrory P, Johnston K, Meeuwisse W, et al. Summary and agreement statement of the Second International Conference on Concussion in Sports, Prague 2004. Physician and Sports Med 2005;33(4):29–40.

[70] Hinton-Bayre AD, Geffen G. Severity of sports-related concussion and neuropsychological test performance. Neurology 2002;59:1068–70.

[71] Saunders RL, Harbaugh RE. The second impact in catastrophic contact: sports head trauma. JAMA 1984;252:538–9.

[72] Cantu RC. Second impact syndrome. Clin Sports Med 1998;17(1):37–44.

[73] Cantu RC, Voy R. Second impact syndrome: a risk in any contact sport. Physician and Sports Med 1995;23:27–34.

[74] McCrory PR, Berkovic SF. Second impact syndrome. Neurology 1998;50(3):677–83.

[75] Kelly JP, Rosenberg JH. Diagnosis and management of concussion in sports. Neurology 1997; 48(3):575–80.

[76] Lovell MR, Collins MW, Iverson GL, et al. Recovery from mild concussion in high school athletes. J Neurosurg 2003;98(2):296–301.

[77] Matser EJT, Kessels AG, Lezak MD, et al. Neuropsychological impairment in amateur soccer players. JAMA 1999;282(10):971–3.

[78] Collins MW, Grindel SH, Lovell MR, et al. Relationship between concussion and neuro-psychological performance in college football players. JAMA 1999;282(10):964–70.

ELSEVIER
SAUNDERS

Pediatr Clin N Am 53 (2006) 27–39

PEDIATRIC CLINICS

OF NORTH AMERICA

Clinical Response to Child Abuse

Mark Hudson, MD*, Rich Kaplan, MSW, MD

Midwest Children's Resource Center, Children's Hospitals and Clinics of Minnesota,
347 North Smith Avenue, Suite 401, St. Paul, MN 55102, USA

The pediatric medical provider is confronted frequently with patients in whom child abuse is a possible concern. It goes without saying that the accurate and timely diagnosis of child maltreatment has the potential to seriously and permanently affect the well being of these children.

Role of the medical provider

Child abuse is a complex phenomenon. Unlike many other conditions evaluated by pediatric practitioners, the diagnosis of child maltreatment requires significant input from nonmedical community sources. The medical provider must form an alliance with community members responsible for the investigation, management, and adjudication of child abuse cases. It is only by collaborating with these team members that a complete clinical picture can be elucidated and diagnosed definitively. Measurements, photographs, and careful descriptions of the scene are often critical to an accurate diagnosis. Likewise, a history from child protection services of previous multiple injuries, previous termination of parental rights, or familial substance abuse may be critical in the assessment of a child's safety and the development of a treatment plan.

The ability to share information with family members may be limited by the possibility that such information could actually put the child at risk for further

* Corresponding author.
E-mail address: Mark.hudson@childrenshc.org (M. Hudson).

0031-3955/06/$ – see front matter © 2006 Elsevier Inc. All rights reserved.
doi:10.1016/j.pcl.2005.09.006

pediatric.theclinics.com

injury. The "family centered care" model may have to be adapted in cases of suspected maltreatment. The role of a medical practitioner in possible child abuse cases requires a keen awareness of the necessity for a team approach, a level of caution in the exchange of information with the family that is not required in other cases, and most of all, a willingness ensure that the diagnosis of child maltreatment is appropriately included in the differential diagnosis.

Abusive head trauma

An association has long been recognized between closed head injury and child abuse. In 1946, an article by Caffey [1] described the association between long bone fractures and chronic subdural hematomas. In this early article, Caffey suggested a whiplash-type mechanism. However, it was not until the 1970s when landmark articles clearly identifying violent acceleration and deceleration as the postulated mechanism were published in refereed medical journals, first in 1971 by Guthkelch and then in 1972 by Caffey [2,3]. From slightly different perspectives, both of these articles noted the relationship among intracranial hemorrhage, child battering, and the lack of evidence of external head trauma. Both authors postulated a mechanism of violent acceleration and deceleration causing a derangement of brain tissue and an injury to cerebral vasculature. From this early research, the concept of the "shaken baby syndrome" (SBS) evolved. Clinicians and scientists alike noted a recurrent constellation of symptoms in victims of abusive head trauma, including intracranial and retinal hemorrhage, evidence of brain injury, and often, characteristic fractures of the ribs and the long bone metaphyses. Over the ensuing decades, this constellation of symptoms became reified into SBS. Recently, many child abuse clinicians and researchers have become somewhat uneasy with the "syndrome" designation and have preferred to describe nonaccidental head injury of infants as abusive head trauma (AHT) or inflicted traumatic brain injury (ie, iTBI). These designations acknowledge the lack of specific observational data and the impracticality of human study. These semantic distinctions in no way diminish the clinical or scientific certainty that this form of abuse does exist.

The incidence of AHT is understandably difficult to measure. Two prospective population-based studies, one in Scotland and one in North Carolina, estimate the incidence at, respectively, 24.6 per 100,000 and 29.7 per 100,000 infants less than 1 year of age. Both studies are well designed, and both face the pitfalls of unidentified and wrongly identified abusive head trauma [4,5]. It is clear from several studies that the risk of abusive head trauma is the highest in children less than 1 year of age. It is important to note that ethnicity has not been shown to be a significant predictor of abusive versus accidental head trauma [6,7].

Four primary pathologic and diagnostic features will be discussed: traumatic injury to the brain substance; causes of intracranial hemorrhage and its diagnostic significance; retinal hemorrhage and its diagnostic significance; and an approach to the evaluation of AHT in the clinical setting.

The precise mechanism of injury to the brain in abusive head trauma has yet to be elucidated clearly. There is general agreement among mainstream clinicians and researchers that the abuse creates shearing forces in the developing infant brain, which cause injury to the axonal system. Symptoms depend on the severity and often include a loss of consciousness, apnea, and cerebral edema. It is this brain substance injury that accounts for the primary symptoms and clinical course of the injured child. This traumatic axonal injury is the key pathologic feature in AHT.

Readily identifiable on radiographic imaging and autopsy, the presence of intracranial blood has long been a central diagnostic feature of AHT. Although axonal injury is the key pathologic feature, the identification of intracranial hemorrhage is certainly important both diagnostically and with respect to medical management. Although subdural hemorrhage is certainly the intracranial pathology most commonly identified in cases of AHT, subarachnoid and epidural hemorrhage have been reported.

Subdural hemorrhage presents typically in one of two forms. First and much more commonly in accidental head trauma is the subdural hemorrhage associated with the translational forces of impact. These contact-type injuries present with clear evidence of impact in the form of soft tissue swelling or actual skull fracture. These are high-force injuries, but a history of accidental impact such as the motor vehicle crash or a fall from a significant height onto a hard surface can be reassuring. The second form is the more diffuse form of subdural hemorrhage resulting from rotational and shearing forces on the bridging veins of the brain surface. Evidence of impact may be present, but there will be diffuse areas of hemorrhage that are often intrahemispheric, all or perifalcial. This form is much less common in infants and suggests AHT.

There is good evidence that accidental subdural hemorrhage in small children is rare. Feldman and colleagues [6] examined a series of children under the age of 3 years and were able to identify nearly 60% who were abused. Interestingly, in Feldman and colleague's study, abuse was much more common in children in whom there was a history of a short fall or no history at all. Delay in seeking care and evidence of other trauma were also significant predictors of abuse. It should be noted that there are multiple studies that have examined the possibility of significant intracranial injury from short and medium distance falls in children. Overwhelmingly, the data reveal that severe injuries resulting from such falls are exceedingly rare and need to be scrutinized carefully [8–12].

Retinal hemorrhages (RH) are frequently noted in abusive head trauma. It is fair to estimate that approximately 80% of children who have suffered abusive head trauma have retinal hemorrhages [13]. There is also good evidence that RH is found more commonly at autopsy than in intact survivors. This certainly suggests that retinal hemorrhaging is a marker of severity [14]. There are case reports of retinal hemorrhages that occur in severe accidental trauma and those that are possibly associated with severe intracranial hypertension [15,16]. In these cases, however, the hemorrhages have been confined to the posterior pole of the retina and have usually been few in number. With increasing knowledge about the variability and pathology RH, it is critically important that a skilled ophthalmologist carefully document the character and location of the hemor-rhage. Markers of severity such as vitreous hemorrhage or retinoschisis should be noted.

The recognition of abusive head trauma is not always straightforward. A 1999 study by Jenny and colleagues [17] has noted that nearly one of three AHT cases were seen by a physician after the abusive episode and were not diagnosed. Reasons for these misdiagnoses included nonspecific presentation by a small infant, absence of external signs of trauma, radiologist error, and the child com-ing from a white, intact, family. This study is not, as it may seem to some, a global indictment of our profession. It is instead a call to strengthen our diag-nostic armamentarium and to encourage all of us to keep child abuse on our dif-ferential diagnoses.

The diagnostic approach to abusive head trauma begins with a careful and well-documented history. Quoted remarks should be used whenever possible, and the child's caregiver should be asked to carefully describe the mechanism of in-jury. The medical provider or child abuse consultant should include in the differ-ential diagnosis any possible medical or accidental causes of the child's symptoms. It is not the physician's role to accuse or confront family members. The medical provider should also refrain from suggesting mechanisms of injury to the family. Finally, it is critically important that the medical care team involve community members of the child abuse team in planning for the safety of the child.

Early consultation with a child abuse pediatrician is critical in planning a diagnostic strategy and providing liaison with community professionals. Deci-sions can be made at that time about other consultations (eg, neurosurgery or ophthalmology or other treatments). Imaging strategies can also be developed in concert with the child abuse consultant. This type of collaboration between hos-pital and community teams will most likely result in the most accurate diagnosis and will minimize trauma to the patient and the patient's family.

Also required for accurate diagnosis is an imaging strategy that addresses the specific radiologic features of AHT, encompassing three primary areas. For head imaging, an initial CT scan is a reasonable place to begin. Although it is not as sensitive as MRI, CT can be obtained quickly and without sedation. CT scanning, however, may miss small extradural blood collections. If there is a high index of suspicion, early MRI may be necessary; otherwise, an MRI study performed during the first 72 hours can be a helpful diagnostic adjunct. This strategy of course should be coordinated with the treatment team. Second, a complete skeletal survey should be undertaken. Using protocols guided by the American College of Radiology, this survey should always be repeated in 2 weeks, when there has been an acute presentation. A nuclear bone scan may be helpful in the first days to identify occult bony injury, but this will not obviate the need for the repeat survey. Special attention should be paid to the ribs and the long bone metaphyses because these fractures are associated commonly with AHT. Finally, with respect to imaging, occult abdominal trauma should be considered. Children with elevated liver function tests or those most likely to have suffered abdominal trauma, toddlers and older infants, should undergo an abdominal CT with contrast if renal function is adequate.

Skeletal injury

Any skeletal injury can be the result of abuse. A careful history evaluated in the context of the patient's developmental stage is the key to differentiating abusive from nonabusive injury. An understanding of the literature surrounding short falls is invaluable. Additionally, some fractures, particularly in infants, should always raise suspicion for abuse.

Household falls in infants are common and usually harmless. A study of more than 11,000 infants less than 6 months of age has revealed that approximately 22% of the infants were involved in a household fall. Less than 1% of these falls resulted in any serious injury (defined as concussion or fracture). There were more than 1700 falls from beds or settees, and only one fracture, a clavicle, was reported [18]. In a second well-designed study, 207 falls ranging in height from 25 to 54 inches occurring in hospitalized children less than 6 years of age resulted in only two fractures, a simple skull fracture and a clavicle fracture [9]. Hennrikus and colleagues [19] report that fractures resulting from falls in children less than 1 year of age were uncommon compared with older children and were injuries of concern for physical abuse in 50% of cases. Even in this study reporting frequent injuries from household falls, the authors urge caution and suggest a careful investigation for nonaccidental trauma when children less than 1 year old present with fractures after a fall from a bed or couch.

Fractures in very young children, particularly nonmobile infants, are often the result of abuse [20,21]. Additionally, there are a few fractures in young children that warrant special attention because of their high specificity for abuse. High-specificity fractures include classic metaphyseal lesions (CML) and rib fractures. Scapular fractures, spinous process fractures, and sternal fractures are also highly specific.

The classic metaphyseal lesion (the corner or "bucket handle" fracture), regardless of history, should be viewed as highly specific for abuse. Until the mid 1980s the CML was believed to be an avulsion fracture at the point of insertion of the periosteum. Kleinman and colleagues [22] studied radiologic and histologic features of these fractures in abused infants at autopsy. Rather than an avulsion fracture, they discovered that the CML is actually a planar series of microfractures through the metaphyseal primary spongiosa. When the lesion is viewed tangentially, a corner fracture appearance is noted. When viewed at an angle, a bucket handle fracture is noted. Coned down views of the metaphyses may be helpful in the evaluation of suspected abuse. In the case of suspected nonaccidental fatal trauma, a postmortem examination of the metaphyses may be indicated even in metaphyses with no radiologic evidence of fracture [23].

Rib fractures, particularly posterior rib fractures, are highly specific for abusive injury in young infants. Although rib fractures have long been known to be highly correlated with abuse, three recent independent case series studies reveal very similar results. In children less than 1, 2, and 3 years of age, 82% to 83% of rib fractures were attributed to abuse. The remaining rib fractures were the result of bone disease or accidental injury. Accidental fractures were rare and were the result of cardiac surgery, pedestrian versus car accidents, motor vehicle crashes, a birth injury, a stairway fall in the arms of the father, and an instance of an older sibling who fell on an infant. In contrast, the fractures attributed to abuse often presented with no history of trauma or a history of minor trauma [24–26]. In two of the studies, abused children were found to have significantly more rib fractures than children with noninflicted injuries, and in 20% to 29%, there were no associated injuries identified [25,26]. Additionally, Cadzow and Armstrong [25] report that one of three children who returned home after an inflicted rib fracture subsequently suffered a significant reinjury.

Cardiopulmonary resuscitation (CPR) is often cited as a cause for rib fractures in critically injured children. This explanation should be viewed with extreme skepticism. Based on the radiologic examination of 50 children who received CPR, Feldman and Brewer [27] report that rib fractures in children are rarely if ever the result of CPR. Spevak and colleagues [28] studied 91 infants who had no evidence of abuse but who had received CPR. These patients were examined both radiologically and on autopsy. No rib fractures were identified.

Posterior rib fractures are the result of unique mechanical forces and are highly suggestive of inflicted trauma. The posterior rib and the transverse process act as a lever mechanism. The transverse process is the fulcrum. As the chest is compressed, the posterior ribs move dorsally, causing excess levering over the transverse process. This injury is typically the result of an adult grasping the child around the chest and squeezing the chest, but it could result from an infant being slammed or hurled face-first into a solid object. This mechanism would also allow chest compression and dorsal migration of the posterior ribs and could be the result of abusive injury or forceful accidental injury such as a motor vehicle crash [29].

Although a discussion of radiologic dating of fractures is beyond the scope of this article, it should be noted that multiple fractures in various stages of healing is an indication of possible abuse.

A skeletal survey is the primary diagnostic tool to identify occult fractures in young children and is mandatory in any child less than 2 years old in whom physical abuse is suspected. A skeletal survey may also be indicated in children 2 to 5 years old based on the history. When abuse is suspected, the skeletal survey should be repeated in 2 weeks. A "babygram" is not acceptable. A skeletal survey should comply with the standards developed by the American College of Radiology. Radionuclide bone scanning may have a role as an adjunct to plain films [30]. Films should be reviewed by a pediatric radiologist.

Cutaneous manifestations of abuse

Bruises are common in children but may be a sign of child abuse. Three factors can assist the clinician in distinguishing inflicted bruises from accidentally acquired bruises: the age and developmental stage of the child, the bruise pattern, and the location.

As with skeletal injury, bruises in young children raise concern for abuse. Sugar and colleagues [31] performed a large prospective cross-sectional survey of children less than 3 years of age who were not suspected to be victims of abuse and had no known medical condition to account for bruises. Only 2.2% of precruisers had any bruises, whereas 17.8% of cruisers and 51.9% of walkers had bruises. Although few precruisers had any bruises, the majority of the bruises in this group were in children greater than 6 months of age. One lesson from this large study is simply stated in the report's title: "Those that don't cruise rarely bruise" [31]. Labbe and colleagues went a step further and examined recent skin injuries in children 0 to 17 years of age. Skin injuries, including bruises, abrasions, scratches, and other injuries, were extremely common in most children. Children 0 to 8 months old, however, had relatively few injuries, and the majority of injuries were scratches on the head and face. Again, bruises were rarely found in this age group (1.2%) [32].

Sometimes being struck with a hand or object results in a patterned bruise or injury. These patterned injuries are seldom the result of routine childhood activity. Some objects leave recognizable patterns. A slow-velocity impact such as a grab or a squeeze may bruise at the points of contact, such as beneath the pads of the assailant's fingers. In this case, capillary disruption occurs directly beneath the force. Conversely, in a high-velocity impact, such as a slap with an open hand, the outline of the fingers may be identifiable as a bruise or petechial injury. In this case, the injury outlines the points of contact, and there is sparing directly beneath the points of contact. A child struck with an object such as a belt may have parallel linear bruises. Again, the injury often outlines the object. A looped cord may leave a "closed loop" imprint on the child's skin. There may even be a laceration of the skin at the tip of the loop. Often, the implement that left the patterned injury cannot be identified by examination alone. Involvement of a multidisciplinary team may allow identification of the implement.

Some pattern injuries are the result of the child's anatomy rather than the implement with which they are struck. Spanking of the buttocks may leave a diagnostic patterned injury consisting of petechial injuries paralleling each side of the gluteal cleft with central sparing. When the child is struck, the buttocks are forced to comply with the shape of the object. As a result, the skin at the margin of the gluteal cleft is forced into an exaggerated fold. Petechial injury occurs along this fold. Bruising of the gluteal convexities may or may not be present. Similarly, an ear that is struck or pinched may have petechae on the edge of the helix, presumably from folding of the helix [33].

Bruise location can offer some insight to the cause. Accidental bruises in mobile children occur most frequently over bony prominences such as shins, knees, and foreheads [31,34,35]. Bruises on the trunk, buttocks, and cheeks are unusual and warrant additional consideration.

Some texts suggest that the color of a bruise can be used to estimate the age of an injury. It is now clear that clinicians cannot accurately predict the age of bruises, and this practice should be avoided [36–38].

All bruises suspected to be inflicted should be photographically documented with a 35-mm format or high-quality digital photographs. Photographs should be taken with adequate lighting and include a measuring device. Multiple photos, including both tight and wide angle, should be obtained.

Inflicted burns are an important manifestation of child abuse. As with all forms of child abuse, an accurate and carefully obtained history is crucial. This history must then be evaluated in the context of the child's development. In scald burns, particular attention should be paid to identifying what the child was wearing at the time of the injury. Hot liquid soaked into clothing in contact with the skin may alter the pattern of a hot liquid burn. The initial physical examination and burn distribution should be carefully documented and photographed if possible. This allows a future review of the injury before medical intervention that may change the appearance of the injury.

Inflicted burns may be the result of contact with hot objects such as cigarettes or curling irons. Patterned burns should raise concern for an inflicted trauma. Inflicted cigarette burns tend to be round, 7 to 8 mm in diameter, and may be multiple, whereas accidental cigarette burns tend to be ill defined. Bilateral symmetric burns (stocking or glove distribution) should raise concern for a forced immersion. A lack of splash marks may indicate that a child was held still, and areas of sparing may give insight into the position of the child at the time of the injury. Spared areas may be the result of the skin being in contact with itself such as in joint flexion or may be the result of the skin being in contact with the fluid receptacle such as the bottom of the bathtub [39].

Abdominal injury

Inflicted abdominal injury is the second leading cause of child abuse fatalities. The fatality rate may be greater than 50% [40]. In young children, abuse is second only to motor vehicle crashes as a cause of abdominal trauma. Independent of comorbid injuries, inflicted abdominal trauma is associated with a sixfold increase in inhospital mortality. Inflicted abdominal injury is often difficult to diagnose. Unlike most cases of accidental abdominal injury, the history is often absent or deliberately falsified. Additionally, this unreliable history may be coupled with vague signs and symptoms. Children with associated fractures may in fact have a lower mortality rate than children without fractures. Presumably, the fractures alert caretakers and medical personnel to the unreported history of trauma [41].

Children with inflicted abdominal injury tend to be younger and present for medical care later than accidentally injured children. Toddlers and young children appear to be at particular risk. Injuries may be the result of punches, kicks, or the child being hurled into other objects. Child abuse can result in either solid- or hollow-organ injury. Any abdominal injury in a toddler or young child without a history of severe trauma such as a motor vehicle crash warrants evaluation. Several studies demonstrate that hollow-organ injury in young children, particularly when reported to be the result of a fall, are injuries of high concern for abuse [40,42]. In fact, fatal blunt force abdominal injury from nonvehicular accidents appears to be so rare that it can almost be viewed as nonexistent [43].

Occult abdominal trauma should be considered in patients with nonspecific signs and symptoms and in patients with other signs of abuse. Abdominal bruising is an important sign, but the absence of bruising does not rule out internal injury because a significant number of patients do not have bruises [42]. Coant and colleagues [44] report a series of patients suspected to have been physically abused who did not have signs or symptoms of abdominal trauma. Four of 49 patients had elevated liver transaminase levels. Three of the four had liver injury documented on CT scan. This suggests that liver enzymes may be a reasonable screen in any patient who is suspected of being abused. In the stable patient, CT is usually the examination of choice and will best demonstrate many of the injuries resulting from abuse [30]. In the opinion of the present authors, the clinician should have a relatively low threshold for obtaining abdominal CT in a patient who has any significant inflicted injury such as AHT or multiple fractures.

Sexual abuse

Child sexual abuse remains a common and vexing problem. A recent study by Finkelhor and colleagues [45] suggests that the prevalence rates for sexual victimization were 96 per 1000 for girls and 67 per 1000 for boys between the ages of 2 and 17 years. Responding to child sexual abuse is often daunting for the pediatric provider. Invariably, the atmosphere is emotionally charged, and the practitioner is faced with a diagnostic and management challenge. In meeting this challenge, it is important to be mindful of the current literature regarding the examination of possible abuse victims as well as some basic principles and procedural guidelines.

It is important to remember that caring for a youngster who may have been sexually abused is, first and foremost, medical care. Although these cases seem unique and the legal aspects may be intimidating, the basic principles of medical care apply. Clinical decision making needs to use the same risk-benefit analysis that the practitioner uses customarily. There may be pressure to perform procedures to facilitate a legal resolution that pose a risk to the patient. Additionally, the emotional state of the child's caregivers, often ranging from terror to rage, may add a sense of urgency to the case.

Because the history and physical evaluation of these youngsters has become so specialized and the potential for emotional trauma so great, these evaluations are best performed in a comfortable, child-friendly setting by practitioners specially trained and facilities specially equipped for such examinations. Therefore, it is critically important that communities develop procedural guidelines to determine what constitutes a true emergency and who will respond if necessary. However, the majority of child sexual abuse cases are not emergent and can be scheduled at a time that is optimum for the comfort of the child and therefore obviate the need for multiple evaluations.

There are times when an urgent evaluation is required. Reasons for emergency examinations include cases of

- Complaints of pain
- Evidence or complaint of bleeding or injury
- An alleged assault that has occurred within the previous 72 hours and the transfer of biologic material may have occurred
- Medical intervention that is needed emergently to assure the safety of the child

With prepubertal children, there is evidence to suggest that forensically significant biologic transfer material rarely lasts longer than 24 hours [46]. These data however, may be updated as modern DNA technology is used. There is still strong evidence, however, that the most likely location of biologic transfer material is in the clothing or bedding related to the assault. Therefore, when assessing the need for and performing an emergency acute sexual assault evaluation, it is critical that community resources be used to obtain clothing and bedding.

Because physical findings are rarely diagnostic in these cases, a well-documented and careful medical history is most often the sole or primary diagnostic evidence. For this reason, obtaining the medical history from an allegedly sexually abused child, sometimes referred to as forensic interviewing, has become a highly specialized practice. Although it is necessary to obtain sufficient information from the child victim to assure their medical well being and safety, it is recommended that the complete and definitive medical history be obtained by a specially trained individual.

In addition to a well-documented history, the alleged child sexual abuse victim needs a thorough physical examination, including a complete physical assessment, looking for other signs of maltreatment and other unrelated medical conditions. It should also include a gentle, well-documented genital examination. Like the history, this genital examination requires special competencies. The ability to provide photographic documentation through video colposcopy or photography is crucial. This documentation will potentially obviate the need for multiple examinations.

There is good evidence that, without specific training, even highly qualified pediatric practitioners are unable to accurately interpret genital findings. In a well-designed study, Makoroff and colleagues [47] note that of 46 nonacute sexual abuse examinations called abnormal by pediatric emergency room physicians, 79% of these examinations were found to be normal or nonspecific by child abuse specialists. These data strongly argue for performing sexual abuse examinations or, at the very least, having the examinations reviewed by trained and experienced child abuse medical providers.

Importantly, the likelihood that nonacute genital examination findings are diagnostic for child sexual abuse is remarkably low. Studies by Berenson and colleagues [48] and Heger and colleagues [49] clearly place the likelihood of diagnostic findings in prepubertal girls, including those who have been penetrated, at less than 5%. Remarkably, an excellent study by Kellogg and colleagues [50] notes normal or nonspecific examinations in pregnant adolescents, a condition that most authors agree has been preceded by sexual contact. The reasons for the lack of clear and definitive findings in these cases are

- The broad range of normal demonstrated in multiple studies [51–53]
- Children's remarkable capacity to heal [54]
- The fact that many disclosures of sexual abuse occur long after the actual trauma
- That many episodes of child sexual abuse, even with penetration, may not be damaging

Finally, when considering child sexual abuse, the pediatric practitioner must be aware that the diagnosis of sexually transmitted infections (STI) has both legal and medical implications. This means that a practitioner must be aware of STI prevalence patterns in the community and region. There has been a shift of late in the probative significance of the various sexually transmitted infections. Children infected with syphilis, gonorrhea, or Chlamydia are still considered to have had sexual contact. However, infections with herpes simplex viruses or human papillomaviruses are increasingly ambiguous with respect to the possibility of a sexually acquired infection. Of course, testing for and, when indicated, prophylaxis against HIV and hepatitis remain critically important measures. A protocol for post-exposure prophylaxis should be available to the practitioner.

Summary

The medical evaluation of child abuse is challenging and requires a highly specialized response. The role of the pediatric medical provider is not significantly different than it is with other unusual or challenging health problems. The child's well being remains the primary concern, and consultation with a child abuse specialist will help to ensure the child's safety.

References

[1] Caffey J. Multiple fractures of the long bones in infants suffering from chronic subdural hematoma. AJR Am J Roentgenol 1946;56:163–73.

[2] Caffey J. On the theory and practice of shaking infants: its potential residual effects of permanent brain damage and mental retardation. Am J Dis Child 1972;124:161–9.

[3] Guthkelch AN. Infantile subdural hematoma and its relationship to whiplash injuries. BMJ 1971;2:430–1.

[4] Barrow K, Minns R. Annual incidence of shaken impact syndrome in young children. Lancet 2000;356:1571–2.

[5] Keenan HT, Runyan DK, Marshall SW, et al. A population-based study of inflicted traumatic brain injury in young children. JAMA 2003;290(5):621–6.

[6] Feldman K, Bethel R, Shugerman R, et al. The cause of infant and toddler subdural hemorrhage: a prospective study. Pediatrics 2001;108:636–46.

[7] Sinal S, Petree A, Hereman-Giddens M, et al. Is race or ethnicity a predictive factor in shaken baby syndrome? Child Abuse Negl 2000;24:1241–6.

[8] Helfer RE, Slovist L, Black M. Injuries resulting when small children fall out of bed. Pediatrics 1977;60:533–5.

[9] Lyons TJ, Oates RK. Falling out of bed: a relatively benign occurrence. Pediatrics 1993;92: 125–7.

[10] Selbst SM, Baker MD, Shames M. Bunk bed injuries. Am J Dis Child 1990;144:721–3.

[11] Joffe M, Ludwig S. Stairway injuries in children. Pediatrics 1988;82:457–61.

[12] Chiavello CT, Bond GR. Stairway-related injuries in children. Pediatrics 1994;94:679–81.

[13] Levin AV. Ocular manifestations of child abuse. In: Reece RM, Ludwig S, editors. Child abuse: medical diagnosis and management. 2nd edition. Philadelphia: Lippincott Williams & Wilkins; 2001. p. 97.

[14] Levin AV. Opthalmic manifestations of inflicted childhood neurotrauma. In: Reece RM, Nicholson CE, editors. Inflicted childhood neurotrauma. Elk Grove Village (IL): American Academy of Pediatrics; 2002. p. 127–63.

[15] Bechtel K, Stoessel K, Leventhal JM, et al. Characteristics that distinguish accidental from abusive injury in hospitalized young children with head trauma. Pediatrics 2004;114:165–8.

[16] Levin AV. Retinal hemorrhage and child abuse. In: David T, editor. Recent advances in pediatrics. London: Churchill Livingstone; 2000. p. 151–219.

[17] Jenny C, Hymel KP, Ritzen A, et al. Analysis of missed cases of abusive head trauma. JAMA 1999;281:621–6.

[18] Warrington SA, Wright CM for the ALPSAC Study Team. Accidents and resulting injuries in premobile infants: data from the ALPSAC study. Arch Dis Child 2001;85:104–7.

[19] Hennrikus WL, Shaw BA, Gerardi JA. Injuries when children reportedly fall from a bed or couch. Clin Orthop 2003;407:148–51.

[20] Blakemore LC, Loder RT, Hensinger RN. Role of intentional abuse in children 1 to 5 years old with isolated femoral shaft fractures. J Pediatr Orthop 1996;16(5):585–8.

[21] Thomas SA, Rosenfield NS, Leventhal JM, et al. Long-bone fractures in young children: distinguishing accidental injuries from child abuse. Pediatrics 1991;88(3):471–6.

[22] Marks SC. The structural and developmental contexts of skeletal injury. In: Kleinman PK, editor. Diagnostic imaging of infant abuse. 2nd edition. St. Louis: Mosby; 1998. p. 9–22.

[23] Kleinman PK, Marks SC, Blackbourne B. The metaphyseal lesion in abused infants: a radiologic-histopathologic study. AJR Am J Roentgenol 1986;146(5):895–905.

[24] Bulloch B, Schubert CJ, Brophy PD, et al. Cause and clinical characteristics of rib fractures in infants. Pediatrics 2000;105(4):E48.

[25] Cadzow SP, Armstrong KL. Rib fractures in infants: red alert! the clinical features, investigations and child protection outcomes. J Paediatr Child Health 2000;36(4):322–6.

[26] Barsness KA, Cha ES, Bensard DD, et al. The positive predictive value of rib fractures as an indicator of nonaccidental trauma in children. J Trauma 2003;54(6):1107–10.

[27] Feldman KW, Brewer DK. Child abuse, cardiopulmonary resuscitation, and rib fractures. Pediatrics 1984;73(3):339–42.

[28] Spevak MR, Kleinman PK, Belanger PL, et al. Cardiopulmonary resuscitation and rib fractures in infants: a postmortem radiologic-pathologic study. JAMA 1994;272(8):617–8.

[29] Kleinman PK, Schlesinger AE. Mechanical factors associated with posterior rib fractures: laboratory and case studies. Pediatr Radiol 1997;27:87–91.
[30] American Academy of Pediatrics, Section on Radiology. Diagnostic imaging of child abuse. Pediatrics 2000;105(6):1345–8.
[31] Sugar NF, Taylor JA, Feldman KW. Bruises in infants and toddlers: those that don't cruise rarely bruise. Arch Pediatr Adolesc Med 1999;153:399–403.
[32] Labbe J, Caouette G. Recent skin injuries in normal children. Pediatrics 2001;108:271–6.
[33] Felman KW. Patterned abusive bruises of the buttocks and pinnae. Pediatrics 1992;90(4):633–6.
[34] Carpenter RF. The prevalence and distribution of bruising in babies. Arch Dis Child 1990;80: 363–6.
[35] Pascoe JM, Hildebrandt HM, Tarrier A, et al. Patterns of skin injury in nonaccidental and accidental injury. Pediatrics 1979;64(2):245–7.
[36] Langlois NE, Gresham GA. The aging of bruises: a review and study of the colour changes with time. Forensic Sci Int 1991;50:227–38.
[37] Stephenson T, Bialis Y. Estimation of the age of bruising. Arch Dis Child 1996;74:53–5.
[38] Bariciak ED, Plint AC, Gaboury I, et al. Dating of bruises in children: an assessment of physician accuracy. Pediatrics 2003;112(4):804–7.
[39] Greenbaum AR, Donne J, Wilson D, et al. Intentional burn injury: an evidence-based, clinical and forensic review. Burns 2004;30:628–42.
[40] Ledbetter DJ, Hatch Jr EI, Feldman KW, et al. Diagnostic and surgical implications of child abuse. Arch Surg 1998;9:1101–5.
[41] Trokel M, DiScala C, Terrin N, et al. Blunt abdominal injury in the young pediatric patient: child abuse and patient outcomes. Child Maltreat 2004;9(1):111–7.
[42] Barnes PM, Norton CM, Dunstan FD, et al. Abdominal injury due to child abuse. Lancet 2005; 366:234–5.
[43] Price EA, Rush LR, Perper JA, et al. Cardiopulmonary resuscitation-related injuries and homicidal blunt abdominal trauma in children. Am J Forensic Med Pathol 2000;21(4):307–10.
[44] Coant PN, Kornberg AE, Brody AS, et al. Markers for occult liver injury in cases of physical abuse in children. Pediatrics 1992;89(2):274–8.
[45] Finkelhor D, Ormord R, Turner H, et al. The victimization of children and youth: a comprehensive national survey. Child Maltreat 2005;10:5–25.
[46] Christian CW, Lavelle JM, De Jong AR, et al. Forensic findings in prepubertal victims of sexual assault. Pediatrics 2000;106:100–4.
[47] Makoroff KL, Brauley JL, Brandner AM, et al. Genital examinations for alleged sexual abuse of prepubertal girls: findings by pediatric emergency medicine physicians compared with child abuse trained physicians. Child Abuse Negl 2002;26:1235–42.
[48] Berenson AB, Chacko MR, Wiemann CM, et al. A case-control study of anatomic changes resulting from sexual abuse. Am J Obstet Gynecol 2000;182:820–34.
[49] Heger A, Ticson L, Velasquez O, et al. Children referred for possible sexual abuse: medical findings in 2384 children. Child Abuse Negl 2002;26:645–59.
[50] Kellogg ND, Menard SW, Santos A. Genital anatomy in pregnant adolescents: "normal" doesn't mean "nothing happened". Pediatrics 2004;223:E67–9.
[51] Berenson AB, Grady JJ. A longitudinal study of hymenal development from 3 to 9 years of age. J Pediatr 2002;140:600–7.
[52] Berenson AB, Heger AH, Hayes JM, et al. Appearance of the hymen in prepubertal girls. Pediatrics 1992;89:387–94.
[53] Adams J, Harper K, Knudson S, et al. Examination findings in legally confirmed cases of child sexual abuse: it's normal to be normal. Pediatrics 1994;94:310–7.
[54] Heppenstall-Heger A, McConnell G, Ticson L, et al. Healing patterns in anogenital injuries: a longitudinal study of injuries associated with sexual abuse, accidental injuries, or genital surgery in the preadolescent child. Pediatrics 2003;112:829–37.

ELSEVIER
SAUNDERS

PEDIATRIC CLINICS

OF NORTH AMERICA

Pediatr Clin N Am 53 (2006) 41–67

Pediatric Upper Extremity Injuries

Sarah Carson, MD[a], Dale P. Woolridge, MD, PhD[a],*,
Jim Colletti, MD[b], Kevin Kilgore, MD[b]

[a]Department of Emergency Medicine, The University of Arizona, 1515 North Campbell Avenue,
Tucson, AZ 85724, USA
[b]Department of Emergency Medicine, Regions Hospital, 640 Jackson Street, St. Paul, MN 55101, USA

The pediatric musculoskeletal system differs greatly from that of an adult. Although these differences diminish with age, they present unique injury patterns and challenges in the diagnosis and treatment of pediatric orthopedic problems.

Pediatric bone is highly cellular and porous, and it contains a large amount of collagen and cartilage compared with adult bone. The larger amount of collagen leads to a reduction of tensile strength and prevents the propagation of fractures, whereas the abundance of cartilage improves resilience but makes radiologic evaluation difficult [1]. The tensile strength of pediatric bone is less than that of the ligaments, so children are more likely to have bone injuries with mechanisms that would cause only ligamentous injuries in adults. The periosteum of pediatric bone is comparatively more metabolically active than the adult periosteum, leading to rapid and large callus formation, rapid union of fractures, and a higher potential for remodeling. The periosteum is also thicker and stronger in children. This difference is responsible for some of the unique fracture patterns seen in children [1,2].

The most obvious difference between the pediatric and the adult skeleton is the presence of growth plates. The physis is a transition zone between the metaphysis and epiphysis. This is a highly metabolic and rapidly changing area of bone. The germinal area of the physis rests on the epiphysis, and cartilage cells grow toward the metaphysis, forming columns of cells. These columns degenerate, undergo hypertrophy, and then calcify at the metaphysis. The growth and change that occur at a growth plate facilitate remodeling of fractures and

---

* Corresponding author.
E-mail address: dale@aemrc.arizona.edu (D.P. Woolridge).

0031-3955/06/$ – see front matter © 2006 Elsevier Inc. All rights reserved.
doi:10.1016/j.pcl.2005.10.003
pediatric.theclinics.com

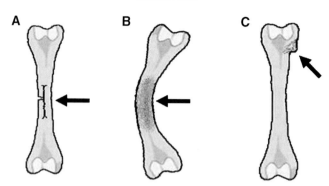

Fig. 1. Pediatric fracture patterns. (*A*) Greenstick fracture demonstrating the direction (*arrow*) of force causing the fracture. Note the fracture line opposite to the side of the force, along with a vertical fracture component. (*B*) Plastic deformity, showing the direction (*arrow*) of force causing the fracture. (*C*) Torus fracture showing the buckle deformity (*arrow*) in the bony cortex.

contribute to rapid healing; however, damage to the physis itself can lead to deformity secondary to asymmetrical growth [3–6].

Fractures in children are less likely to propagate and become comminuted. Greenstick fractures, common in the forearm, illustrate this well. The bone bends before it breaks, but because of the thick outer portion of the bone, the periosteal sleeve maintains apposition and creates a "hinge" effect (Fig. 1A) [2,7]. In some cases, the periosteum may remain completely intact, and the bone may be bowed, which is known as a plastic deformity. It is common in the forearm as well, and it is likely seen in conjunction with another fracture (see Fig. 1B). Torus, or buckle fractures, are also a result of the high collagen content of pediatric bone. The bone is more likely to fail in both tension and compression. This fracture is commonly seen in the distal radius (see Fig. 1C) [7].

Physeal injuries

Physeal injuries are unique to children, and they account for approximately one fourth of all pediatric fractures. Although a majority of these fractures heal without incidence, approximately 30% of these fractures cause a growth disturbance, and 2% of them cause a functional growth deformity. A number of classification systems exist for these fractures, but the Salter-Harris classification system is the simplest and most widely used. Salter-Harris type I injury is a fracture through the hypertrophic cartilage that causes a widening of the physeal space. These fractures are difficult to diagnose radiographically and are clinically hallmarked by point tenderness at the epiphyseal plate (Fig. 2). Type II fractures are the most common. These extend through both the physis and metaphysis. Although these fractures may result in some shortening, they rarely cause functional deformities (see Fig. 2). Type III injuries extend through the physis

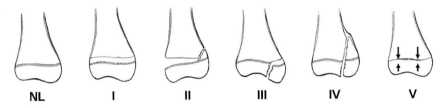

Fig. 2. Salter-Harris (SH) fracture types. NL, normal physis; I, type I fracture through the pelvis; II, type II fracture through the physis and metaphysis; III, type III fracture through the physis and epiphysis; IV, type IV fracture through the physis, metaphysis, and epiphysis; V, type V fracture showing a crush injury (*arrows*) of the physis.

and the epiphysis, disrupting the reproductive layer of the physis. These injuries may cause chronic sequelae because they disrupt the articular surface of the bone, but they rarely cause any deformity and generally have a good prognosis (see Fig. 2). Type IV injuries cross through all three areas of bone, the epiphysis, physis, and metaphysis. These fractures are also intra-articular, increasing the risk for chronic disability. They also can disrupt the proliferative zone, leading to early fusion and growth deformity. Type V fractures are the least common but most difficult to diagnosis and have the worst prognosis. The classic mechanism on injury is an axial force that compresses the epiphyseal plate without an overt fracture of the epiphysis or metaphysis. Although a type V Salter-Harris fracture may not be radiographically apparent, radiographs may demonstrate a joint effusion. This compressive mechanism results in premature closure of the physis and thereby arresting bone growth [3,4,8]. Type V injuries are commonly diagnosed in retrospect, secondary to the occult nature of the radiograph.

Evaluation

Proper injury management is contingent on the correct diagnosis. The evaluation of the child may be complicated by other injuries and the lack of cooperation on the part of the child. It is vital to obtain an accurate history, including the situation, mechanism, and timing of the injury. The orthopedic physical examination follows the standard sequence of inspection, palpation, range of motion, and neurovascular examination. First, observe the patient for any obvious deformity and watch for spontaneous movement. Lack of spontaneous movement may be true paralysis, but pseudoparalysis is common in children who have had trauma or infection. It is important to remove all splints, bandages, and obscuring clothing to perform an accurate examination. Look for any breaks in the skin, deformity, swelling, or ecchymosis. Depending on the ability of the patient to cooperate, have the patient locate the point of maximal tenderness. This is vital to the correct diagnosis in some cases because the presence of unossified bone makes some fractures difficult to diagnose. Palpate the entire limb, including the joint above and below the obvious injury. It is also important to remember the shoulder, clavicle, and scapula when performing an upper extremity orthopedic examination. Evaluate both the passive and active ranges of motion of the entire extremity. With an uncooperative patient, this may be difficult. Finally, it is important to assess the neurovascular status of the patient. For the vascular examination, the presence of a pulse alone is not an adequate test of circulation. The capillary refill rate is a more sensitive test of perfusion. Observe while the patient passively extends the fingers. Pain with this activity may be an early sign of ischemia. A complete neurologic examination of both sensory and motor functions of the extremity is an important part of the assessment, as well.

Imaging

Although the history and physical examination are important in the correct diagnosis, a majority of orthopedic injuries are diagnosed with radiographic imaging. Conventional radiography is adequate to diagnose a majority of injuries, but some injuries may require additional views or other imaging modalities. It is necessary to obtain at least two views of the injured area, and as it is important to carefully examine the joint above and below the injury, because these areas may require imaging as well. The presence of ossification centers can make radiographic evaluation difficult, especially of the wrist and elbow. It may be helpful to obtain films of the uninjured extremity for comparison. Difficulty with radiographic evaluation can often occur in young infants, whose bones have not begun to ossify at the site of interest. In these cases, ultrasonography or CT scanning may be needed to further elucidate the injury. With these imaging modalities, cartilaginous structures and associated effusions can be better appreciated [8,9].

Consultation

It is important when consulting a specialist to accurately describe the injury, including severity, location, description of the fracture line, displacement, separation or shortening, angulation, and any complicating findings from the physical examination, including delayed capillary refill or neurologic deficits. If there is a fracture, note first whether it is open or closed. Virtually all open fractures, with the exception of open distal phalanx fractures, require urgent operative management and immediate orthopedic consultation. The location of the injury includes not only the bone involved but also whether the injury is proximal, distal, or midshaft and whether there is involvement of the articular surface. The fracture line describes the defect in the bone. The line may be linear or spiral. There also may be more than one fracture line. Fractures that have more that one line and break the bone in many pieces are comminuted. Two separate fractures that result in a free-floating segment of bone are segmental. Displacement implies that the two fracture fragments are offset from each other. It may be described in measured distance or a percentage of the width of the proximal piece. The direction of displacement can be described as volar, dorsal, anterior, posterior, radial, ulnar, medial, or lateral. Separation is the distance that the distal segment is removed from the proximal segment. Shortening is the distance that the bone has been shortened as a result of either impaction or an over-riding fracture fragment. Angulation defines the angle that the distal fragment takes in relation to the proximal fragment. It is easily determined by noting the number of degrees that the distal fragment would need to be rotated to be parallel to the proximal fragment. If any neurologic deficit or vascular compromise is noted, an orthopedist should be consulted [10].

Traumatic injuries by location

Clavicle

The clavicle is one of the bones most frequently broken in children, although most fractures heal well with minimal or no treatment [11,12]. Clavicle fractures may occur in newborns, caused by compression of the shoulders during birth. In children and adolescents, fractures typically occur from a fall on an outstretched arm or shoulder. Fractures may also be the result of a direct blow, accounting for the majority of distal clavicle fractures. In infants and young children, these fractures are typically greenstick fractures and may go unnoticed until a large callus forms [12]. In older children, the fracture is usually displaced completely, resulting in a lowering of the affected shoulder, local swelling, and tenderness. Pediatric clavicle fractures rarely require operative treatment. An asymptomatic fracture in the newborn and infants may be treated with "benign neglect," and parents are cautioned to handle the child carefully. In infants with a significant amount of pain, the arm may be splinted for 7 to 14 days. Midshaft clavicle fracture in children and adolescents are treated with a sling or a figure-of-eight bandage, which is worn for 1 to 4 weeks for comfort only. Fractures are only reduced if the integrity of the overlying skin is in jeopardy [12,13].

True dislocations of the clavicle are rare in children and are more often physeal injuries. Medial physeal injuries may be displaced anteriorly or posteriorly. The patient typically has pain and swelling at the medial end of the clavicle. Severe posterior dislocation can cause compression of the trachea, subclavian vessel, or brachial plexus [11]. Lateral physeal separation presents clinically as pain with all movements of the shoulder. Depending on the severity of the injury and degree of displacement, the skin may be tented over the acromioclavicular joint. Treatment of medial injuries is usually conservative if there is no evidence of mediastinal injury or significant cosmetic deformity, and patients are treated symptomatically with a sling or a figure-of-eight harness. A closed reduction is attempted for more serious medial injuries [11,14]. Minor lateral physeal injuries with minimal displacement are treated symptomatically with a sling, but more severely displaced injuries typically require open reduction.

Scapula

Scapular fractures are rare and are usually the result of high-energy trauma. They are usually associated with other injuries, including clavicle fracture, rib fracture, pneumothoraces, thoracic vertebral fractures, and fractures of the humerus. The diagnosis of scapular fracture is often delayed because of these associated injuries. Treatment is often conservative, with patient comfort being the goal of treatment. Most patients tolerate a sling or shoulder immobilizer and are able to perform gentle range of motion exercise after 2 weeks. Complications are not common and are generally related to malunion or associated thoracic injuries.

Shoulder

Dislocations of the shoulder are rare in infants but more common in adolescents [15]. In the young child, proximal humeral injuries consist of a fracture at the physis. These fractures account for approximately 3% to 7% of all physeal injuries [16]. Difficulty can arise when evaluating a young infants' shoulder because the humeral head is primarily cartilaginous. In such an event, radiography will not be able to distinguish between a physeal fracture and a dislocation. In this case, ultrasonography or MRI imaging is of benefit. Proximal physeal fractures occur in children of any age but are most common in adolescents. These fractures may result from a fall on an outstretched arm or from a direct blow, with the former being more common. Infants may sustain these fractures as a result of birth trauma or child abuse. On physical examination, there is localized swelling and tenderness, and the affected arm may be shortened and held in abduction and extension. There also may be distortion of the anterior axillary fold. Proximal humeral physeal injuries are almost exclusively Salter-Harris type I and II and have the potential for significant remodeling. The treatment of these fractures is generally nonoperative, even with significant displacement. A sling, sling and swath, or shoulder immobilizer is worn until pain subsides. Two weeks after the injury, the patient may begin pendulum exercises. Most patients resume some overhead activities within 4 to 6 weeks. Complications are rare; however, the most common complication is shortening of the humerus secondary to physeal damage and growth retardation [16–18].

Shoulder dislocation

The glenohumeral joint is one of the most flexible joints the body, but this flexibility is achieved at the expense of stability. There is little bony stability of the shoulder. Both static and dynamic supports are provided almost solely by muscles and ligaments. Traumatic dislocations of the shoulder are typically the result of indirect force. Greater than 90% of dislocations are anterior dislocations, but posterior and inferior dislocations do occur. Traumatic dislocations are acutely painful. With anterior dislocations, the arm is held in abduction with external rotation. The humeral head may be palpable anteriorly, and there is a palpable defect just inferior to the acromion. Posterior dislocations are rarer, accounting for less than 3% of these injuries, and they are more commonly missed [11]. The arm is usually held in adduction with slight internal rotation. The shoulder may also appear flat anteriorly with a prominent coracoid process. Luxio erecta, or inferior dislocation, is the rarest traumatic dislocation. The arm is maximally abducted and adjacent to the head. These injuries can occur with enough force to drive the humeral head through the axilla, creating an open injury. Shoulder dislocations are commonly diagnosed by physical examination, but the diagnosis should be confirmed radiologically, along with any noted associated fractures. A thorough neurovascular examination should be performed. Special attention should be paid to the axillary nerve because it is most commonly injured with anterior dislocations. Acute shoulder dislocations should be reduced as quickly as possible. There are many techniques for reducing these injuries. Anterior shoulder dislocations are commonly reduced under procedural sedation with a traction–counter-traction technique. If an assistant is not available to provide counter-traction, there are many modifications of this technique. For instance, the patient is mildly sedated and placed in a prone position with the affected limb dangling over the edge of the bed. With enough time, the shoulder will reduce. Radiographs should be obtained after reduction to confirm anatomic placement as well as to look for any traumatic fracture. The neurovascular examination should be repeated. The patient is usually placed in a sling for comfort and can resume full activity within 2 to 3 weeks [15,19]. The most common complication of these injuries is recurrent instability. The incidence of recurrent dislocations has been reported to be as high as 70% to 90% [14]. These injuries may also be complicated by a fracture of the glenoid fossa or humeral head (the Hill-Sachs lesion), neurovascular injuries, and osteonecrosis of the humeral head [11,19,20].

Humerus

Fractures of the humeral metaphysis are more common in children than in adolescents, because adolescents are more likely to have a humeral physeal fracture [11]. Most of these fractures are caused by a high-energy direct blow to the metaphysis, and they are often associated with multiple traumas [21]. Any fracture to this area with a history of minimal trauma should raise the suspicion of a pathologic fracture or abuse. The humerus is a common location of bone cysts and other benign lesions [21]. These injuries typically present with localized pain, deformity, and swelling. Evaluation of the radial nerve is imperative because it is vulnerable to these fractures. Injury to this nerve will cause numbness to the dorsum of the hand between the first and second metacarpal and loss of strength with thumb and wrist extension and forearm supination. Humeral shaft fractures are the second most common birth fracture. Neonates with this injury are treated with immobilization of the arm next to the thorax for 1 to 3 weeks, and a follow-up examination is required to exclude a brachial plexus injury. These fractures, like humeral physeal fractures, have a high potential for remodeling. Patients are treated with a coaptation splint for 2 to 3 weeks and then treated in a sling or hanging arm cast [22]. It is not necessary to achieve end-to-end alignment of these fractures. Angulation greater than 15° to 20° or any rotational deformity needs to be addressed by a specialist. Complications are rare, with radial nerve injury being the most frequent.

Supracondylar fracture

Epidemiology

Supracondylar fractures occur most commonly between 3 and 10 years of age, with a peak incidence at age 5 to 7 and a mean age of 7.9 years [23–25]. Overall, these fractures are the most common pediatric elbow fracture, accounting for over half of all elbow fractures in children and a third of pediatric limb fractures [23]. For this reason, the following sections focus on this fracture type.

There are two major classifications of supracondylar fracture, extension and flexion. Extension fractures account for approximately 95% of supracondylar fractures. The mechanism of injury of a supracondylar extension fracture is a fall on an outstretched hand (FOOSH) with the elbow hyperextended (eg, a fall from the playground "monkey bars"). The FOOSH mechanism causes the ulna and triceps muscles to exert an unopposed force on the distal humerus, thereby resulting in posterior displacement of the fracture [25]. This extension mechanism results in a shift of the condylar complex in either the posterolateral or the posteromedial direction. Supracondylar flexion fractures account for 5% of supracondylar fractures. They occur secondary to a direct blow to the posterior aspect of the flexed elbow and result in anterolateral displacement of the condylar complex [26].

Clinical presentation

The child with a supracondylar fracture presents with swelling at the elbow and localized tenderness; and with a supracondylar extension fracture, the child presents with a proximal depression over the triceps. The physical examination should focus on the degree of swelling and neurovascular status. Excessive swelling and ecchymosis at the elbow are concerning signs of extensive soft tissue injury, which is a significant risk factor for compartment syndrome [27]. It is critical that the clinician perform a thorough neurovascular assessment. Neurovascular evaluation includes palpation of the distal pulses and assessment of skin color, temperature, capillary refill, and the sensory and motor aspects of the median, radial, and ulnar nerves. If a pulse is not detected by palpation, examination by Doppler ultrasound should be undertaken. A concerning sign of ischemia is increasing pain or pain with passive extension of the fingers [24]. In the presence of ischemia, an orthopedic surgeon must be consulted immediately to evaluate and reduce the fracture. In cases of supracondylar extension fractures, the examination should focus on assessment of the brachial artery as well as the median and radial nerves.

Radiographic findings

Radiographs should be obtained in children who present with a clinical presentation suggesting a supracondylar fracture, an unclear history, or localized tenderness or swelling of the elbow. Both an anteroposterior view in extension and a lateral view at 90° of flexion should be undertaken. As the pediatric radiograph are interpreted, consideration should be given to the stages of ossification. Radiographs should be assessed for fracture lines and, if present, the degree of fracture displacement and angulation. Because fracture lines are often difficult to visualize, attention should also focused on the subtle signs of a supracondylar fracture such as the presence of fat pads, the anterior humeral line, and the absence of the figure-of-eight.

Interpretation of the pediatric elbow radiograph is challenging secondary to the different stages of ossification [25]. The first ossification center, the capitellum, appears at approximately 1 year of age followed by the radial head at roughly 3 years of age. The third site to appear is the medial or internal epicondyle at roughly 5 years of age, followed by the trochlea at roughly 7 years. The final two ossification centers are the olecranon (approximately 9 years of age) and the lateral or external epicondyle (approximately 11 years of age). A helpful memory aid for recalling the radiographic order of ossification sites of the pediatric elbow is the acronym CRITOE (*c*apitellum, *r*adial head, *i*nternal epicondyle, *t*rochlea, *o*lecranon, *e*xternal epicondyle), remembering that the capitellum appears at 1 year of age and each ossification site in the mnemonic appears in a 2-year progression (ie, 1, 3, 5, 7, 9, and 11 years).

The radiograph of the elbow should be assessed for the presence of fat pads, the anterior humeral line, and the figure-of-eight at the distal humerus. Fat pads are a nonspecific marker of hemorrhage or an elbow joint effusion. Depending on the location and size of a fat pad, it may be an indicator of an occult fracture. An anterior fat pad can be a normal variant when it is seen as a narrow radiolucent strip superior to the radial head and anterior to the distal humerus. If the anterior fat pad is wide, it is known as a "sail" sign and is indicative of a fracture, but a small anterior fat pad may be normal. The posterior fat pad results from visualization of fat from the olecranon fossa. It appears radiographically as a radiolucency posterior to the distal humerus and adjacent to the olecranon fossa. The presence of a posterior fat pad is never normal and is indicative of pathology. As such, the radiographic presence of a posterior fat pad requires careful immobilization and close follow-up.

The anterior humeral line is a line drawn through the anterior cortex of the humerus that intersects the capitellum in its middle third. In the presence of a posteriorly displaced supracondylar fracture, the anterior humeral line passes through the anterior third of the capitellum, or it may entirely miss the capitellum. An assessment of the figure-of-eight requires a true lateral view. Disruption of the figure-of-eight indicates a supracondylar fracture.

Management

Immediate therapy consists of pain management, application of a splint for comfort, and elevation of the arm above the level of the heart. Further management is determined by the classification of supracondylar fracture based on radiographic findings. There are three classifications of supracondylar fractures. Type I is a nondisplaced fracture suspected either on clinical grounds or radiographically by the presence of the sail sign or posterior fat pad (Fig. 3). The child may be discharged home if the family is perceived as reliable, able to assess neurovascular status, and live close to the hospital. The child should be placed in a posterior splint from the wrist to the axilla, with the elbow at 90° of flexion and the forearm in its neutral position for at least 3 weeks [24]. It is advisable to avoid circumferential casting and extremes of flexion in an effort to decrease the incidence of compartment syndrome and vascular compromise [25,28]. If a child meets criteria for discharge, the family should be instructed to return immediately for signs of unmanageable pain or the child's inability to extend his or her fingers. For the discharged child, close orthopedic follow-up (within 24 hours) must be established. Type II supracondylar fractures are angulated and displaced fractures in which the posterior cortex remains intact

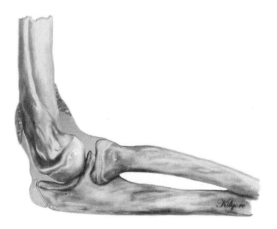

Fig. 3. Salter-Harris type I nondisplaced fracture.

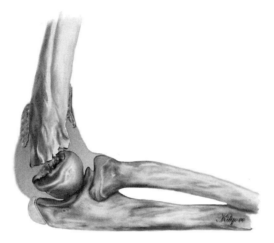

Fig. 4. Salter-Harris type II supracondylar fractures are angulated and displaced fractures in which the posterior cortex remains intact.

(Fig. 4). Type II fractures require a pediatric orthopedic evaluation. The choice of therapy, for example, closed ED reduction versus percutaneous pinning, is based on the degree of deformity as well as the adequacy and stability of the fracture reduction. The child should be immobilized in a noncircumferential splint at 110° of flexion. All children with type II posteriorly displaced supracondylar fractures should be admitted to the hospital for neurovascular assessment secondary to the increased probability of neurovascular compromise. Type III fractures have a disrupted posterior periosteum with a completely displaced distal fragment, without contact between fragments (Fig. 5). Type III fractures may be displaced

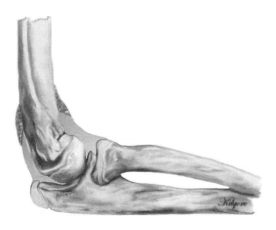

Fig. 5. Salter-Harris type III fractures have a disrupted posterior periosteum with a completely displaced distal fragment, without contact between fragments.

in three directions: posteromedial (the most common pattern), posterolateral, or anterolateral. The direction of displacement is important in determining which neurovascular structures may be injured (see complications in the following section). All type III supracondylar fractures require orthopedic consultation for the evaluation of closed or open reduction with percutaneous pin placement, hospitalization for vigilant neurovascular assessments, and close follow-up.

The flexion type of supracondylar fracture results from a direct force to the posterior elbow, resulting in anterior displacement of the distal segment and disruption of the posterior periosteum. A pediatric orthopedist should be consulted promptly, and these children require hospitalization for frequent neurovascular assessment. Immediate reduction should be attempted in cases in which there is neurovascular compromise and orthopedic consultation is not available.

Complications

Complications of supracondylar fractures include nerve injury, vascular compromise (brachial artery), forearm compartment syndrome resulting in Volkmann's ischemic contracture, and loss of range of motion.

Overall the incidence of supracondylar-associated neurovascular injury is 12% and increases with displacement to between 19% and 49% [29–31]. Nerve function before fracture reduction should be documented. The most commonly injured nerve is arguably the median (28%–60%), followed closely by the radial (26%–61%), and then the ulnar (11%–15%) nerves [30–32]. Median nerve injury occurs most commonly from posterolateral displacement and results in weakness of the flexor muscles of the hand and loss of two-point sensation in the index and middle fingers [33]. The anterior interosseous nerve is the branch of the median nerve most commonly injured [25,31,33]. Injury to the anterior interosseous nerve is difficult to detect because it lacks a superficial sensory component. Motor impairment is manifested by impairment of the flexor digitalis profundus to the index finger and the flexor pollicis longus as well as mild weakness in supination [25,34]. The motor aspect of the anterior interosseous nerve can be examined by asking the patient to flex the interphalangeal joint of the thumb against resistance or have the patient make an okay sign and assess strength [25,33]. Injury to the radial nerve occurs from posteromedial displacement of the fracture. Anterior displacement of the supracondylar flexion fracture may have an associated ulnar nerve injury. Although nerve injuries may be associated with long-term sequelae, the majority are neurapraxias and will resolve in time [25,30,33,35,36]. Most of these injuries resolve within 2 to 3 months, but in some instances, it may take up to 4 to 5 months for function to return [25,30,33, 35,36].

The absence of the radial pulse is reported in 7% to 12% of all supracondylar fractures and up to 19% of displaced fractures [26]. The brachial artery is injured most commonly in posterolaterally displaced fractures [26]. Vascular injury can lead to compartment syndrome, with associated necrosis and fibrosis of the involved musculature. Compartment syndrome of the volar forearm may develop within 12 to 24 hours [24]. Suspected compartment syndrome should indicate making compartment pressure measurements and immediate consultation with a pediatric orthopedist. When a diagnosis of compartment syndrome is confirmed by compartment measurement, a fasciotomy procedure is indicated [25]. If a compartment syndrome is untreated, the associated ischemia and infarction may progress to the feared complication of Volkmann's ischemic contracture. Volkmann's ischemic contracture is characterized by fixed flexion of the elbow, pronation of the forearm, flexion at the wrist, and joint extension of the metacarpal-phalangeal joint [24].

Cubitus varus or "gunstock" deformity is a common long-term complication of a supracondylar fracture [36]. Cubitus varus occurs when a supracondylar fracture heals with a varus deformity. Overall it is more of a cosmetic issue than one of function.

Transphyseal fractures

Transphyseal fractures are most common in children under 2 years of age. In younger children, these fractures are a result of rotary of shear force, whereas in older children, the fracture is usually caused by a fall on an outstretched hand. Transphyseal fractures are difficult to distinguish radiographically from elbow dislocations [37]. With transphyseal fractures, however, the relationship of the radial head and capitellum is preserved, whereas with dislocations, it is disrupted. In children under the age of 2, in whom the capitellum has not yet ossified, these fractures are even more difficult to diagnose. These fractures are managed by obtaining an acceptable reduction and maintaining it until the fractures heals. These fractures may simply be splinted after reduction, but there is an increased incidence of cubitus varus, and they may be managed by closed reduction and percutaneous pinning [37]. In patients, this fracture is the result of abuse in up to 50% of cases, and the most serious potential complication is not recognizing the abuse and returning the child to a dangerous environment [37]. In older children, the mechanism of transphyseal fractures is similar to that of supracondylar fractures, and the complications are similar, except that neurovascular injury is not common as it is with supracondylar fractures [37,38].

Lateral condyle fractures

Fractures of the lateral condyle of the humerus are typically the result of a fall on an outstretched arm. The lateral condyle is either avulsed by varus stress or displaced by the radial head under valgus stress [39]. Children with these fractures complain of pain and decreased range of motion. In patients with minimally displaced fractures, localized lateral tenderness may be noted. The most common radiographic finding is the presence of a posteriorly displaced metaphyseal fragment known as the Thurston-Holland fragment. The fracture line may also extend to involve the capitellum. These fractures may be difficult to distinguish from transphyseal fractures. Lateral condyle fractures disrupt the anatomic relationship between the radial head and the capitellum, whereas with transphyseal fractures, it is maintained [39,40]. Minimally displaced fractures may not be evident, and oblique views may be helpful. Lateral condyle fractures are all transphyseal and intra-articular, and most require open reduction and internal fixation [39,40]. Complications include cubitus varus, formation of lateral spurs, delayed union, nonunion, and growth arrest [39].

Medial epicondyle fractures

Medial epicondyle fractures account for up to 12% of pediatric elbow fractures and are associated with elbow dislocations up to 50% of the time [41]. They are most common in children 7 to 15 years of age. The medial epicondyle is the insertion point of the ulnar collateral ligament and the flexor muscles of the forearm. Valgus stress produces traction on the medial epicondyle through the flexor muscles. The child typically holds the elbow in flexion, and any movement is painful. There is point tenderness over the medial epicondyle [41,42]. Ulnar nerve paresis and dysthesias may be present because of its close proximity. The medial epicondylar fragment is usually visualized on plain radiograph in older children (those over the age of 6 or 7) with this injury. The fragment may be trapped in the joint space, especially if there is an associated dislocation [42]. Comparison views may be helpful to assess for medial joint space widening in younger patients in whom the medial epicondyle has not yet ossified. Minimally displaced fractures are managed conservatively in a long arm splint or cast for 1 to 2 weeks, with early range of motion exercises to follow. Fractures displaced more than 5 mm may be managed either operatively or conservatively. If the fracture fragment is intra-articular, the fragment must be removed, and this is performed most commonly by surgery. The most common complications are stiffness, ulnar nerve injury, and symptomatic nonunion. Stiffness is avoided by short-term immobilization (less than 3 weeks) and early range of motion exercise. Ulnar nerve injuries occur in 10% to 16% of these fractures, but injury is more likely if the fracture fragment in trapped in the joint [41,42].

Elbow dislocations

Elbow dislocations are not common in the pediatric population, and there are often associated fractures about the elbow, including the medial epicondyle, proximal radius, olecranon, and coranoid process [42–44]. These injuries are seen in adolescents, and the presence of an elbow dislocation in a younger patient should raise the suspicion for a transphyseal fracture [37]. The mechanism of injury is frequently a fall on an outstretched hand. Posterior dislocations are most common, but anterior, medial, lateral, and divergent dislocations can occur. The direction of displacement depends on the force applied. Posterior dislocations are the result of a fall onto an extended or partially flexed supinated forearm. Anterior dislocations result from a direct blow, such as a fall on the olecranon process. Medial and lateral dislocations are secondary to direct trauma or twisting of the forearm. Divergent dislocations are exceeding rare and result in the ulna and radius being displaced in opposite directions [43]. Physical findings include a painful, swollen elbow held in flexion with a seemingly shortened forearm and longer upper arm. Any attempts of movement are painful. All radiographs should be examined carefully for associated fractures. A thorough neurovascular examination is important because the anatomic relationships of the brachial artery, median nerve, and ulnar nerve make them vulnerable. These dislocations are managed generally with procedural sedation and closed reduction. For posterior dislocations, the arm is hyperextend while traction is applied to disengage the forearm and restore length. The elbow is then gently flexed while maintaining traction [43]. Anterior dislocations are frequently associated with extensive soft tissue damage. They are reduced by longitudinal traction being applied to flexed forearm. The elbow is then gently extended as firm pressure is applied distally and posteriorly. The arm is then immobilized in a long arm splint. Radiography after reduction is imperative, and these patients are typically hospitalized for observation because compartment syndrome has been reported after elbow dislocations. Patients are immobilized for 1 to 2 weeks, after which time active range of motion is encouraged to prevent stiffness. Stiffness is the most common complication of elbow dislocation but can be avoided with the appropriate immobilization and institution of range of motion activities. Myositis ossificans and heterotopic bone have also been reported. Vascular injury is not common except with open injuries. Nerve injury patterns mimic those seen with fractures about the elbow and are more common than vascular injuries. The ulnar nerve is the most commonly injured nerve and is associated with medial epicondyle fracture [42]. Median nerve injury also occurs, but it is more difficult to diagnose because of the delayed appearance of motor and sensory symptoms.

Radial head and neck fractures

In children, the radial head is composed of cartilage and is resistant to fracture. As a result, children are more likely to fracture the radial neck. These fractures are rarely isolated because they are associated with other injuries about the elbow, approximately 50% of the time [45]. The radial head or neck may be broken by a fall on an outstretched hand with the elbow in extension and valgus. This mechanism may also cause a fracture of the medial epicondyle, olecranon, proximal ulna, or lateral condyle or rupture of the medial collateral ligament. Elbow dislocation may also fracture the radial neck. With posterior dislocations, the radial head abuts the capitellum. Force at the time of injury or the time of spontaneous reduction may fracture the radial neck. The radial head may be fractured with anterior elbow dislocations, as well [43]. These injuries do not have remarkable physical findings because there is rarely any visible deformity. Children may have some localized swelling and tenderness over the lateral aspect of the elbow. There is pain with passive flexion and extension, but patients experience more pain with pronation and supination of the forearm. Fractures of the radial head and neck may be subtle. If this fracture is suspected, radiographs of the proximal radius should be obtained in addition to elbow films. These fractures are classified by the degree of angulation. Type I injuries have less than 30° of angulation, type II have thirty to 60° of angulation, and type III injuries have more than 60° of angulation [46]. Type I injuries can be managed simply with a sling or posterior splint or long arm cast for 1 to 2 weeks. Closed reduction is attempted in children older than 10 years of age with any angulation greater than 15° because of their decrease potential for remodeling. Type II and III injuries are reduced with procedural sedation [46,47]. If a suitable closed reduction (less than 30° of angulation) cannot be obtained, percutaneous or intramedullary reduction is performed. The most common complication of these injuries is loss of joint motion, specifically rotation. This loss of motion is more likely with severely displaced fractures, other associated elbow injuries, patients older than 10 years of age, any delay in diagnosis or treatment, and substandard reductions. Avascular necrosis may develop after radial head fractures because of the unique blood supply of the radial head. It is estimated that between 10% and 20% of radial neck fractures result in avascular necrosis (AVN), resulting in a clinically significant loss of movement [47].

Olecranon fractures

Olecranon fractures account for only 5% to 7% of all elbow fractures. An association with other elbow injuries is seen in up to half of these fractures [44]. The olecranon is protected from serious injury in children because, in younger children, it is cartilaginous, and the relatively thick periosteum in older children leads to minimally displaced greenstick fractures [7]. Many mechanisms may result in this type of fracture, including hyperextension, hyperflexion, direct blow to a flexed elbow, or a shear force. Physical findings include a swollen tender elbow and possible abrasion or contusion over the olecranon. Radiographs should be examined carefully for other injuries, because these are common. Fractures with a displacement of 3 mm or less are managed conservatively with 3 to 4 weeks of cast immobilization. Fractures that are extra-articular with more than 3 mm of displacement are managed with closed reduction and cast immobilization [44,45]. The position of immobilization is dependent upon the mechanism. Hyperextension and shear injuries are usually stable if they are immobilized in flexion, whereas flexion injuries are most stable in extension. Intra-articular fractures require open reduction and internal fixation [44]. The most serious complication of these fractures is the failure to recognize a concomitant injury, but delayed and nonunion peripheral nerve injury and compartment syndrome have all been reported [44].

Rare elbow fractures

T-condylar fractures are rare in children and are usually the result of a high-energy injury. With these fractures, the medial and lateral columns of the humerus separate from each other and the humeral shaft. With minimal displacement and no comminution, these fractures may be managed with closed reduction and percutaneous pinning, but more serious injuries require open reduction and internal fixation. T-condylar fractures are complicated by stiffness, nonunion and AVN of the trochlea [48].

Medial condyle fractures are not as common as lateral condyle fractures, but they mimic lateral condyle fractures radiographically and clinically. The management and the associated complications of these injuries are similar [48]. The capitellum is rarely fractured in young children because it is still cartilaginous. This injury is seen almost exclusively in adolescents. Because this fracture is intra-articular, it requires open reduction and internal fixation [48].

Radial head subluxation

Radial head subluxation, or "nursemaids' elbow," is produced by traction on the hand with the elbow extended and the forearm pronated. It is the most common upper extremity injury in children under 6 years of age, with peak incidence between 1 and 3 years of age [49,50]. The radial head is oval in shape. With the forearm in supination, the anterior aspect of the radial head is elevated. Traction causes the bony prominence to be pulled next to the annular ligament. With the forearm in pronation, the anterior aspect of the radial head is more rounded, and traction allows the radial head to slip under the annular ligament. As children age, the annular ligament becomes thicker and has stronger distal attachments, thus explaining the age distribution of this injury. The diagnosis is made by history and physical examination. Classically, the child cries immediately after having traction force applied to an outstretched arm [50]. The arm is held in slight flexion with the forearm pronated. The child usually refuses to use the arm. There is usually no visible swelling or deformity. Radiographic findings are normal and are not required with an accurate history [49]. Classically, reduction is achieved by gripping the effected elbow and, with the opposite hand, supinating the wrist and then flexing the elbow. An alternative method is to grip the effected elbow and, with the opposite hand, hyperpronating the forearm. It has been demonstrated that the success rate for reduction with supination is between 80.4% and 92%; however, the hyperpronation has been shown to have a rate as high as 97.5% and has been successful when the supination-flexion technique failed [50] The child will usually begin using the arm again within minutes. Parents should be cautioned that recurrence rate is as ranges from 26.7% to 39%, and they should avoid pulling on the child's hand [50]. If the subluxation has been present for more than 24 hours, closed reduction may not bring any relief, and the child may be placed in a long arm splint. There has also been evidence that shows that reduction attempted less than 2 hours after the injury may be less effective. Without a history suggestive of subluxation of the radial head, radiographs may be obtained to exclude fracture or joint infection.

Forearm fractures

Fractures of the shaft of the radius or ulna account for 10% to 45% of pediatric fractures [51–55]. These injuries vary greatly because they may involve one or both bones and may be complete, and up to 50% of them are greenstick fractures [54]. Complete fractures of the forearm have the potential to be significantly displaced and angulated, with overriding fracture fragments. Plastic deformities are also commonly seen in the forearm [56]. Forearm fractures are usually treated successfully with closed reduction because of the substantial remodeling potential of pediatric bone [5,54,57]. Forearm fractures are usually the result of a fall on an outstretched hand, but direct trauma of significant force can cause both bone forearm fractures, as well [54,58]. Direct trauma to the forearm can result in an ulnar shaft fracture, known as a "nightstick" injury. Patients with fractures of the distal one third, which are more common, present with the classic "dinner fork" deformity [54]. Swelling, deformity, and point tenderness are seen with displaced fractures, but plastic deformity, greenstick, and buckle fractures may have more subtle findings on physical examination. It is not usual for these patients to present days after the original injury occurs. The skin requires careful examination for any in-to-out puncture injury because this injury requires immediate orthopedic consultation and operative treatment. It is essential that at least two radiographic views be obtained to determine an accurate measurement of displacement and angulation. If only one bone is fractured, radiographs of the wrist and elbow should be obtained to exclude a Galeazzi or Monteggia fracture (discussed below) [54].

A Monteggia fracture is a fracture of the proximal third of the ulna with an associated radial head dislocation [54,59,60]. These fractures are clinically significant because of the complications that can arise from these injuries. The radial head is in close anatomic proximity to both the radial and median nerves, causing nerve palsies with dislocation of the radial head. Compartment syndrome can also be seen [59,60]. Patients with this injury usually present with an obvious deformity of the elbow and forearm. The radial head may be palpated, displaced from its usual anatomic location. The skin should be examined carefully for any sign of an open fracture, and a thorough neurologic examination should be performed, with special attention paid to the posterior interosseous nerve. Radiographs of the elbow should be obtained with any isolated fracture of the ulna. Fractures that are diagnosed and treated acutely can be managed successfully with closed reduction and cast immobilization. Operative intervention is required when an adequate closed reduction cannot be obtained or maintained. If the diagnosis is overlooked, the child may develop a chronic or missed Monteggia fracture [60,61]. Complications of treated fractures include recurrent radial head dislocation, malunion, posterior interosseous nerve palsy, and Volkmann's ischemic contracture [62].

With the exception of physeal and distal metaphyseal fractures and Monteggia and Galeazzi fractures (discussed below), forearm fractures are classified according to completeness, location, and direction of angulation. Radial and ulnar shaft fractures usually have good outcomes when treated with closed reduction and cast immobilization [52,54,57]. Operative treatment is required for open fractures, arterial injuries, irreducible fractures, failed reductions, and skeletal maturity. Refracture is the most common complication of these injuries and occurs in 7% to 17% of forearm fractures [54]. It is more likely following a greenstick or open fracture. Delayed union and nonunion are rare and are associated with open injuries with significant bone or soft tissue loss [53]. Synostosis may occur as a result of high-energy trauma or surgical manipulation, but it is rare in the pediatric population. Compartment syndrome may also occur and may be caused by any casting placed [54]. If a full cast is placed at the time of injury, it should be split to allow for swelling. If there is any suspicion of compartment syndrome, including pain with extension of the digits, paresthesia, pallor, or lack of pulse, the cast should immediately be split to the skin or removed altogether. The radial, median, and ulnar nerves are all susceptible to injury with forearm fractures. Injury to the anterior interosseous nerve is seen with fractures of the radius [54]. Nerve injury can occur at the time of injury or during a closed reduction. If possible, a complete neurologic examination should be performed before reduction, although this is sometimes difficult with the pediatric patient.

Distal forearm fractures

Distal forearm fractures are common in children, and they account for 75% to 84% of pediatric forearm fractures [51,54]. They include buckle or torus, greenstick, metaphyseal, physeal, and Galeazzi fractures. These fractures are also typically the result of a fall on an outstretched hand. Displacement of the fracture depends on the position of the wrist at the time of the injury. A fall on a dorsiflexed wrist will result in a dorsally displaced fracture, with the converse being true. Buckle or torus fractures are more common with low-energy injuries, whereas displaced fractures are seen following higher energy mechanisms. The patient may have a "dinner fork" deformity, but physical findings may be subtle. A careful examination of the wrist and elbow should be performed to look for any associated injuries. As with all fractures of the forearm, careful skin and neurologic examinations are imperative. Physeal fractures are classified according to the Salter-Harris classification system. Isolated radius fractures should raise the suspicion of a Galeazzi fracture, which is a fracture of the distal radius with associated disruption of the radioulnar joint [52,63,64].

Buckle fractures are usually managed successfully in short arm casts [51]. This provides comfort and prevents any further displacement. It is important to note the involvement of the physis as the time of injury. If the physis is involved, it must be reevaluated in 6 to 12 months.

Greenstick fractures are managed with closed reduction and long arm casting. Although there is controversy regarding the position of the forearm during immobilization, the neutral position is accepted widely as the most appropriate position [48,51]. These fractures heal quickly and well, and the cast is removed after 6 weeks. Parents must be cautioned about the possibility of reinjury [54,55,57,58].

Forearm metaphyseal fractures usually involve both bones. The radius is usually involved as a complete fracture, and the ulna may have a complete, greenstick, styloid avulsion fracture, or a plastic deformity. Typically, the goal of treatment is to ensure adequate reduction of the radius, and this in turn, usually results in good results with any involved ulnar fractures [54–57]. Nondisplaced fractures are immobilized in a cast for 4 weeks. Displaced fractures are treated with closed reduction and casting for 4 to 6 weeks. The indications for operative management include open fractures, reductions that are not adequate or cannot be maintained, fractures associated with compartment syndrome or carpal tunnel syndrome, fractures with severe swelling, and those with ipsilateral fractures requiring stabilization (usually supracondylar fractures) [48,53,54].

Fractures of the distal radial physis can be managed with closed reduction and casting. These fractures heal quickly, requiring only 3 to 4 weeks of immobilization, and have a high potential for remodeling [5,6,51] Fractures presenting more than 3 days after the original injury should not be reduced because there is an increased likelihood of damaging the physis [48]. All Salter-Harris III and IV fractures require open reduction because they are, by definition, intra-articular fractures.

The distal ulnar physis is only rarely fractured, and there is controversy regarding the optimal way to manage these fractures. Some studies indicate that growth arrest with these injuries is common; however open reduction has not been shown to decrease the incidence of growth arrest [48]. Fortunately, growth arrest of the distal ulna only rarely causes any significant clinical or cosmetic symptoms. Fractures of the ulnar styloid are common and are seen with approximately one third of distal radius fractures. An avulsed ulnar styloid typically requires no treatment and results in an asymptomatic nonunion [54].

Galeazzi fractures are fractures of the distal radius with disruption of the radioulnar joint. Children may have separation of the ulnar physis instead of true disruption of the radioulnar join [63,64]. This is known as a Galeazzi-equivalent injury. Both true Galeazzi fractures and Galeazzi-equivalent injuries can be managed usually with closed reduction in younger children. The goal of treatment is do prevent proximal migration of the distal radial fragment and stabilization of the radioulnar joint. Older children, like adults, require an open reduction [52,54,62–64].

Pediatric distal forearm fractures generally have a good prognosis. Malunion is the most frequent complication, although it is not usually symptomatic for the patient. Other complications may include refracture, growth arrest, nerve injury, and compartment syndrome.

Wrist and hand

The carpus is composed entirely of cartilage at birth and remains predominantly cartilaginous until the late childhood and adolescent years. As a result, mechanisms that would produce bony wrist injuries in the mature skeleton produce fractures of the forearm bones in young children. The capitate is the first carpal bone to begin ossification at 2 to 3 months of age, and the hamate closely follows approximately 1 month later. Ossification then proceeds in a clockwise manner. The triquetrum begins to ossify at 2 years of age, the lunate ossifies at age 3, the scaphoid ossifies at age 5, and the trapezoid and trapezium ossify at age 6. The pisiform does not appear on radiographs until 9 or 10 years of age. Carpal fractures in younger children, although rare, are usually associated with other fractures [65]. Adolescents have patterns of injury similar to adults. Although not common, ligamentous injuries may be associated with carpal fractures in children [65]. These injuries can cause lasting sequelae, including stiffness and weakness, and require prompt identification and treatment.

As in adults, the scaphoid is the carpal bone most commonly fractured in children [48,66]. The typical patient is an adolescent male who fell on an outstretched arm. These fractures may be associated with ligamentous injuries. Clinically, the patient has radial-side wrist pain, mild swelling in the anatomic "snuff box," and tenderness directly over the scaphoid. Both swelling and tenderness should be compared with the unaffected wrist. Scaphoid fractures often have subtle findings on radiographs, and there is no imaging modality to accurately assess for any ligamentous injury. If there is suspicion of a scaphoid fracture, the wrist must be immobilized in a short thumb spica cast, and repeat radiographs should be obtained 14 to 21 days later. Plain radiographs should include a dedicated scaphoid view and comparison views. If the repeat radiographs are negative but the patient continues to be symptomatic, CT scans, bone scans, and MRI are all suitable alternative imaging modalities to visualize an occult fracture [48]. Nondisplaced fractures are treated with a short thumb spica cast for 4 to 8 weeks. Any displacement on radiographs is a sign of instability and warrants open reduction and internal fixation. Adolescent athletes may have nondisplaced fractures repaired operatively to assure stability and to allow earlier return to activity [66].

Wrist dislocation and fracture-dislocation

Wrist dislocations and subluxations are exceedingly difficult to diagnosis in children. The wrist is unossified, making radiographs difficult to interpret. A dislocation or subluxation must be ruled out when a child presents with a painful, swollen wrist that is unable to flex or extend and no forearm fracture is evident. Comparison views are essential in the diagnosis. These rare injuries usually require additional imaging with arthrography or MRI to better delineate the nature of the injury [48,65,67].

Hand fractures

Pediatric hand fractures are rarely complicated injuries and are usually treated adequately with splinting or casting. Open reduction is required for fractures that fail closed reduction. Single metacarpal fractures only require splinting and protection while healing; however multiple metacarpal fractures are usually unstable and may require pinning. Additionally, any metacarpal fracture with rotational deformity significant enough to cause finger overlap usually requires open reduction [67,68]. Severely angulated proximal and middle phalanx fractures or displaced intra-articular fractures require open reduction. All other fractures may simply be managed with closed reduction, if necessary, and splinting [67–71]. The distal phalanx is closely associated with the nail bed. A significant fracture of this bone is commonly associated with nail trauma, which requires repair. Conversely, any significant nail trauma should be imaged to look for an underlying fracture. Fractures that are not significantly displaced, although they are technically open fractures, do not require immediate orthopedic consultation. The patient may be treated with oral antibiotics, splinting, and orthopedic follow-up [68].

Hand infections

Pediatric hand infections are not as common as in adults. The most common infections are those of the fingertip, paronychia, felons, herpetic whitlow, and infections following trauma.

Paronychia is infection of the paronychial tissue. It may be either acute or chronic. It is usually the result of a pulled "hangnail," and it is characterized by redness, swelling, and tenderness at the lateral edge of the nail plate. There is a potential for the infection to course along the bottom edge of the nail. If the infectious process continues, it may undermine the nail plate itself. Causative organisms are *Staphylococcus aureus* and oral anaerobes. Acute paronychias are treated with warm soaks, elevation, and antibiotics. Persistent paronychia with purulent tissue is elevation of the nail fold, or if the infection has already loosened the nail plate, it is removed. Antibiotic coverage should include *S aureus* and oral flora. Chronic paronychias are rarely seen in children, and mixed flora, including fungi, infection should be suspected [72,73].

A felon is an infection of the pulp space in the distal segment of the finger. Felon infections usually follow penetrating trauma. Clinically, they are characterized by intense pain, erythema, and swelling of the palmar aspect of the distal phalanx. *S aureus* is the most common organism identified. Treatment includes antibiotics covering this organism and surgical drainage of the infection. The septae of the pulp space are divided, and a wick is placed for 48 hours [72,73].

Herpetic whitlow is a superficial skin infection of the herpes simplex virus. In children, it is almost exclusively caused by the oral herpesvirus, herpes simplex virus I. Prodromal symptoms are pain and tingling over the effected area. Vesicles will later appear. The vesicles are initially clear on an erythematous base, giving the typical "dewdrops on a rose petal" appearance. Vesicles later become cloudy because of cellular response. The infection is self-limiting and resolves in 5 to 7 days. Care should be taken to prevent spreading by covering the area. Treatment is symptomatic and includes analgesia. Oral acyclovir may shorten the course of the infection if given early in the prodromal phase. Topical acyclovir is not effective. Repeated whitlows may be an indication of immune compromise [74].

Pyogenic tenosynovitis is infection of the tenosynovium within the flexor tendon sheaths. This space is closed and causes predictable spreading of the infection. This infection is characterized by Kanavel's signs: fusiform swelling of the finger, tenderness over the flexor sheath, pain with passive extension of the finger, and the finger held in flexion. The infection manifests 12 to 24 hours after penetrating trauma. *S aureus* is the most frequent infecting organism. Treatment is elevation, intravenous antibiotics, and repeat evaluation in 12 to 24 hours. If symptoms and signs persist, a surgical incision and drainage procedure is indicated [75].

Deep space infections include infections in the thenar and midpalmar space. The hand is usually swollen and erythematous, with a globular appearance. These infections are secondary to penetrating trauma, with *S aureus* being the most common causative organism. Treatment is the same as for pyogenic tenosynovitis, and complications include skin necrosis, tendon rupture, and stiffness. Children may become systemically ill with these infections and appear toxic [68,73].

Neonatal brachial plexus injury

Neonatal brachial plexus palsy occurs because of birth trauma. The incidence of neonatal brachial plexus palsy has declined because of improved obstetric practices. This injury results from traction forces applied to the arm, which stretches or tears the brachial plexus. Risk factors include shoulder dystocia, high birth weight, cephalopelvic disproportion, breech position, and prolonged labor [76,77].

Brachial plexus injury is classified by the level of nerve involvement and the nature of the injury. The nerve palsies have been categorized by the level of involvement. Type I injury, or Erb's palsy, involves C4–6 nerve roots. Type II injury, or Erb-DuChenne-Klumpke, involves the entire brachial plexus. Type III, or Klumpke palsy, involves only C8–TI. Mild injuries are stretch injuries of C5–6. Clinically, it manifests with elbow extension, forearm pronation with active motion of the hand. These injuries generally have a good prognosis with recovery of function within 3 months. Moderate injury involves C5–7. The elbow is held in slight flexion, the forearm is adducted, and the hand is loose. Moderate injuries involve avulsion of some nerve roots and simply stretching of others [73]. The recovery of function is slow and incomplete. Maximal function is usually observed within 2 years. Severe injuries involve avulsion of nerve roots C5–T1. These patients have abducted arms, flaccid limbs with the wrist flexed, and the hand held in a claw position. Severe injuries have a poor prognosis, and these patients typically have no recovery of function [76]. Concomitant injuries or deformities that increase suspicion of brachial plexus nerve palsy include Horner syndrome, paralysis of the diaphragm, clavicle fracture, humeral fracture, traumatic shoulder dislocation, spasticity of the lower limbs or opposite upper limb, and hip dysplasia-dislocation [73].

Neonates may have other birth injuries that mimic brachial plexus palsy. Pseudoparalysis because of fracture of the clavicle, humeral physis, or humeral shaft may clinically resemble the deformities noted with these nerve injuries. Osteomyelitis or septic arthritis of the shoulder should also be included in the differential diagnosis. Any treatment is aimed at residual disabilities. Common disabilities include a loss of external rotation and abduction and shoulder dislocation.

Summary

The pediatric musculoskeletal system differs greatly from that of an adult. Although these differences diminish with age, they present unique injury patterns and challenges in the diagnosis and treatment of pediatric orthopedic problems. The differences in physical and chemical makeup of the bone, periosteum, and the presence of growth plates result in an injury pattern and complication pattern that is unique to the pediatric skeleton. Likewise, the evaluation of the child may be complicated by other injuries and the child's lack of cooperation. The orthopedic physical examination follows the standard sequence of evaluation but requires basic knowledge of pediatric injury patterns and treatment. For this reason, the evaluation of orthopedic injuries in children requires a unique approach.

References

[1] Frost HM, Schonau E. "The muscle-bone unit" in children and adolescents: a 2000 overview. J Pediatr Endocrinol Metab 2000;13:571–90.
[2] Specker BL, Brazerol W, Tsang RC, et al. Bone mineral content in children 1 to 6 years of age. Am J Dis Child 1987;141:343–4.
[3] Iannotti JP. Growth plate physiology and pathology. Orthop Clin North Am 1990;21:1–17.
[4] Mizuta T, Benson WM, Foster BK, et al. Statistical analysis of the incidence of physeal injuries. J Pediatr Orthop 1987;7:518–23.
[5] Johari AN. Remodeling of forearm fractures. J Pediatr Orthop Part B 1999;8:84–7.
[6] Murray DW, Wilson-MacDonald J, Morscher E, et al. Bone growth and remodeling after fracture. J Bone Joint Surg Br 1996;78B:42–50.
[7] Jacobson FS. Periosteum: its relation to pediatric fractures. JPO-B 1997;6:84–90.
[8] Salter RB, Harris WR. Injuries involving the growth plate. J Bone Joint Surg Am 1963;45:587.
[9] Kissoon N, Galpin R, Gayle M, et al. Evaluation of the role of comparison radiographs in the diagnosis of traumatic elbow injuries. J Pediatr Orthop 1995;15:449–53.
[10] Schultz RJ. The language of fractures. Baltimore (MD): Williams & Wilkins; 1990.
[11] Bishop JY. Pediatric shoulder trauma. Clin Orthop 2005;432:41–8.
[12] Kubiak R, Slongo T. Operative treatment of clavicle fractures in children: a review of 21 years. J Pediatr Orthop 2002;22:736–9.
[13] Wilkes JA, Hoffer MM. Clavicle fractures in head-injured children. J Orthop Trauma 1987; 1:55.
[14] Lewonowski K, Bassett GS. Complete posterior sternoclavicular epiphyseal separation: a case report and review of the literature. Clin Orthop 1992;281:84–8.
[15] Deitch J, Mehlman CT, Foad SL, et al. Traumatic anterior shoulder dislocation in adolescents. Am J Sports Med 2003;31:758–63.
[16] Robinson CM, Aderinto J. Posterior shoulder dislocation and fracture-dislocation. J Bone Joint Surg Am 2005;87A:639–50.
[17] Baxter MP, McIntyre W, Wiley J. Fracture of the proximal humeral epiphysis: their influence on humeral growth. J Bone Joint Surg Br 1986;68B:570–3.
[18] Neer CS, Horowitz BS. Fractures of the proximal humeral epiphyseal plate. Orthopedics 1965; 41:24–31.
[19] Hovelius L, Augustini G, Fredin O, et al. Primary anterior dislocation of the shoulder in young patients. J Bone Joint Surg Am 1996;78A:1677–86.
[20] Rowe C. Prognosis in dislocation of the shoulder. J Bone Joint Surg Am 1984;38A:957–77.
[21] Shaw BA, Murphy KM, Shaw A, et al. Humerus shaft fractures in young children: accident or abuse? J Pediatr Orthop 1997;17:293–7.
[22] Cartner MJ. Immobilization of fracture of the shaft of the humerus. Injury 1973;5:175.
[23] Della-Giustina K, Della-Giustina DA. Emergency department evaluation and treatment of Pediatric orthopedic injuries. Emerg Med Clin North Am 1999;17:895–922.
[24] Wu J, Perron AD, Miller MD, et al. Orthopedic pitfalls in the ED: pediatric supracondylar humerus fractures. Am J Emerg Med 2002;20:544–9.
[25] Villarin LA, Beck KE, Freid R. Emergency department evaluation and treatment of elbow and forearm injuries. Emerg Med Clin North Am 1999;17:844–58.
[26] Skaggs D, Pershad J. Pediatric elbow trauma. Pediatr Emerg Care 1997;13(6):425–34.
[27] Simon RR, Koeingsknecht SJ, editors. Emergency orthopedics: the extremities. Stamford (CT): Appleton & Lange; 1987. p. 122–9.
[28] McGraw JJ, Akbarnia BA, Hanel DP, et al. Neurological complications resulting from supracondylar fractures of the humerus in children. J Pediatr Orthop 1986;6(6):647–50.
[29] Campbell CC, Waters PM, Emans JB, et al. Neurovascular injury and displacement in type III supracondylar humerus fractures. J Pediatr Ortho 1995;15(1):47–52.
[30] Lyons ST, Quinn M, Stanitski CL. Neurovascular injuries in type III humeral supracondylar fractures in children. Clin Orthop 2000;376:62–7.

[31] Brown IC, Zinar DM. Traumatic and iatrogenic neurological complications after supracondylar humerus fractures in children. J Pediatr Orthop 1995;15(4):440–3.

[32] Heras J, Duran D, de la Cerda J, et al. Supracondylar fractures of the humerus in children. Clin Orthop 2005;432:57–64.

[33] Jones ET, Louis DS. Median nerve injuries associated with supracondylar fractures of the humerus in children. Clin Orthop 1980;150:181–6.

[34] Pirone AM, Graham HK, Krajbich JI. Management of displaced extension type supracondylar fractures of the humerus in children. J Bone Joint Surg Am 1988;70A:641–51.

[35] Ippolito E, Caterinie R, Scola E. Supracondylar fractures of the humerus in children. J Bone Joint Surg Am 1986;68A:333–44.

[36] Lins R, Sinovitch R, Water P. Pediatric elbow trauma. Orthop Clin North Am 1999;30(1):119–32.

[37] Abe M, Ishizu T, Nagaoka T, et al. Epiphyseal separation of distal humeral epiphysis: a follow-up note. J Pediatr Orthop 1995;15:426–34.

[38] deJager LT, Hoffman EB. Fracture-separation of distal humeral epiphysis. J Bone Joint Surg Br 1991;73B:143–6.

[39] Mirsky EC, Karas IG, Weiner CS. Lateral condylar fracture in children: evaluation of classification and treatment. J Orthop Trauma 1997;11:117–20.

[40] Bast SC, Hoffer MM, Aval S. Nonoperative treatment for minimally and nondisplaced lateral humeral condyle fractures in children. J Pediatr Orthop 1998;18:448–50.

[41] Farsetti P, Potenza V, Caterini R, et al. Long-term results of treatment of fractures of the medial humeral epicondyle in children. J Bone Joint Surg Am 2001;83A:1299–305.

[42] Fowles JV, Slimane N, Kassab MT. Elbow dislocation with avulsion of medial humeral epicondyle. J Bone Joint Surg Br 1990;72B:102–4.

[43] Carlioz H, Abols Y. Posterior dislocation of the elbow in children. J Pediatr Orthop 1984;4:8–12.

[44] Graves SC, Canale ST. Fracture of the olecranon in children: long-term follow-up. J Pediatr Orthop 1993;13:239–41.

[45] Dormans JP, Rang M. Fracture of the olecranon and radial neck in children. Orthop Clin North Am 1990;21:257–68.

[46] Leung AG, Peterson HA. Fracture of radial head and neck in children with emphasis on those that involve articular cartilage. J Pediatr Orthop 2000;20:7–14.

[47] Evans MC, Graham HK. Radial neck fractures in children: a management algorithm. J Pediatr Orthop 1999;8(Suppl B):93–9.

[48] Herring JA, Tachdjian MO, editors. Tachdjian's pediatric orthopedics. 3rd edition. Philadelphia: WB Saunders; 2002. p. 2115–252.

[49] Macias CG, et al. History and radiographic findings associated with clinically suspected radial head subluxations. Pediatr Emerg Care 2000;16:22–5.

[50] Macias CG, Bothner J, Wiebe R. A comparison of supination/flexion to hyperpronation in the reduction of radial head subluxations. Pediatrics 1998;102:10–4.

[51] Boyer BA, Overton B, Schrader W, et al. Position of immobilization for pediatric forearm fractures. J Pediatr Orthop 2002;22:185–7.

[52] Jones K, Weiner DS. The management of forearm fractures in children: a plea for conservatism. J Pediatr Orthop 1999;19:811–25.

[53] Luhmann SJ, Schootman M, Schoenecker PL, et al. Complication and outcomes of open pediatric forearm fractures. J Pediatr Orthop 2004;24:1–6.

[54] Rodriguez-Merchan EC. Pediatric fractures of the forearm. Clin Orthop 2005;432:65–72.

[55] Schimittenbecher PP. State-of-the-art treatment of forearm shaft fractures. Injury 2005;36(Suppl A): S25–34.

[56] Borden S. Traumatic bowing of the forearm in children. J Bone Joint Surg Am 1974;56A:611–6.

[57] Blount WP. Forearm fractures in children. Clin Orthop 2005;423:4–7.

[58] Vorlat P, De Boeck H. Bowing fractures of the forearm in children: a long-term followup. Clin Orthop 2003;413:233–7.

[59] Karachalios T, Smith EJ, Pearse MF. Monteggia equivalent injury in a very young patient. Injury 1992;23:419–20.

[60] Papvasiliou VA, Nenopoulos SP. Monteggia-type elbow fracture in childhood. Clin Orthop 1988;233:230–3.
[61] Reckling FW. Unstable fracture-dislocations of the forearm (Monteggia and Galeazzi lesions). J Bone Joint Surg Am 1982;64A:857–63.
[62] Stein F, Grabias SL, Deffer PA. Nerve injuries complicating Monteggia lesions. J Bone Joint Surg Am 1983;53A:1432–6.
[63] Kraus B, Horne G. Galeazzi fractures. J Trauma 1985;25:1903–5.
[64] Landfried MJ, Stenclik M, Susi JG. Variant of Galeazzi fracture-dislocation in children. J Pediatr Orthop 1991;11:332–5.
[65] Light TR. Injury to the immature carpus. Hand Clin 1988;4:415–24.
[66] Wuff RN, Schmidt TL. Carpal fractures in children. J Pediatr Orthop 1998;18:462–5.
[67] Campbell Jr RM. Operative treatment of fractures and dislocation of the hand and wrist region in children. Orthop Clin North Am 1990;21:217–43.
[68] Bhende MS, Dandrea LA, Davis HW. Hand injuries in children presenting to the emergency department. Ann Emerg Med 1993;22:1519–23.
[69] Stahl S, Jupiter JB. Salter-Harris III and IV epiphyseal fractures in the hand treated with tension-band wiring. J Pediatr Orthop 1999;19:233–5.
[70] Fischer MD, McElfresh EC. Physeal and periphyseal injuries of the hand: patterns of injury and results or treatment. Hand Clin 1994;10:287–301.
[71] Torre BA. Epiphyseal injuries in the small joints of the hand. Hand Clin 1988;4:411–21.
[72] Jebson PJ. Infections of the fingertip: paronychias and felons. Hand Clin 1998;14:547–55.
[73] Staheli LT, editor. Practice of pediatric orthopedics. New York: Lippincott Williams & Wilkins; 2001. p. 203–61.
[74] Walker LG, Simmons BP, Lovallo JL. Pediatric herpetic hand infections. J Hand Surg Am 1990;15:176–80.
[75] Jeffrey Jr RB, Laing FC, Schechter WP, et al. Acute suppurative tenosynovitis of the hand: diagnosis with ultrasound. Radiology 1987;162:741.
[76] Noetzel MJ, Wolpaw JR. Emerging concepts in the pathophysiology of recovery from neonatal brachial plexus injury. Neurology 2000;55:5–6.
[77] Lindell-Iwan HL. Obstetric brachial plexus palsy. J Pediatr Orthop 1998;5:210–5.

PEDIATRIC CLINICS

OF NORTH AMERICA

Pediatr Clin N Am 53 (2006) 69–84

Newborn Emergencies: The First 30 Days of Life

Tonia Brousseau, DO[a],*,
Ghazala Q. Sharieff, MD, FACEP, FAAEM, FAAP[b]

[a]*Wolfson Children's Hospital, 955 Yacht Harbor Court, Jacksonville, FL 32225, USA*
[b]*Children's Hospital and Health Center, University of California, San Diego, San Diego, CA, USA*

The evaluation and appropriate management of the critically ill neonate (≤ 28 days of age) require an intimate knowledge of the physiologic changes and life-threatening pathologic conditions that may present during this time. The innate differences in this fragile population may provoke anxiety for the emergency department (ED) physician. For this reason, a broad systematic approach to evaluating the neonate is necessary to provide a comprehensive yet specific differential diagnosis for a presenting complaint or symptom. The efficient recognition and prompt management of illness in the neonatal period may be life saving. In recent years, it has become more important for the ED physician to be familiar with the neonate because of early discharge policies from newborn nurseries. This review provides a systematic approach to the recognition, emergency stabilization, and management of the more common newborn emergencies.

Neurologic emergencies

Recognizing a neurologic insult in neonates may be difficult. The clinical symptoms may be nonspecific. The history may reveal only a change in feeding pattern or subtle behavioral changes. A useful mnemonic to recall the broad differential diagnosis of a neonate with altered mental status, "THE MISFITS," is outlined in Box 1. Keeping this mnemonic in mind as well as a high index of suspicion during the initial history and physical examination (non) will help guide the evaluation and management.

* Corresponding author.
E-mail address: tbrousseau@hotmail.com (T. Brousseau).

Box 1. Causes of altered mental status in a neonate: THE MISFITS

T–Trauma (nonaccidental and accidental)
H–Heart disease and hypovolemia
E–Endocrine (eg, congenital adrenal hyperplasia and thyrotoxicosis)
M–Metabolic (electrolyte imbalance)
I–Inborn errors of metabolism
S–Sepsis (eg, meningitis, pneumonia, and urinary tract infection)
F–Formula mishaps (eg, under- or overdilution)
I–Intestinal catastrophes (eg, volvulus, intussusception, and
   necrotizing enterocolitis)
T–Toxins and poisons
S–Seizures

Seizures

Seizures occurring during the neonatal period are often difficult to recognize. The cortical development is not complete, and as a result, generalized motor activity is less common. Subtle seizures in the term neonate can include abnormal eye movements (usually horizontal, sustained eye deviation), lip smacking, abnormal tongue movements, pedaling, or apnea [1,2].

Although hypoxic-ischemic events are the more common cause of neonatal seizures (60%), the list of other causes is extensive [3]. Box 2 provides the different causes of neonatal seizures based on the age of presentation. Because intracranial infections account for 5% to 10% of neonatal seizures, a thorough sepsis evaluation should be completed on all neonates in the absence of any other immediately apparent cause.

The initial evaluation should include stabilizing the airway, breathing, and circulation (ABC) and obtaining the blood glucose level. The correction of hypoglycemia ($\leq$40 mg/dL) should be accomplished with a 10% dextrose solution, 2 to 4 mL/kg intravenous (IV) [4]. While obtaining vascular access, additional blood tests should include serum electrolytes, a complete blood count (CBC), and blood culture. Lorazepam, 0.1 mg/kg IV, is the initial drug of choice in neonatal seizures [4]. Lorazepam is considered superior to diazepam because of the smaller volume of distribution and longer half-life [5]. If the seizure continues then phenobarbital should be the second-line choice, followed by phenytoin or fosphenytoin. Table 1 includes the pharmacologic management and doses of antiepileptic medications for status epilepticus in the neonatal period.

Other electrolyte imbalances that can result in seizures include hypocalcemia and hyponatremia. Hypocalcemia ($\leq$7 mg/dL) should also be corrected with 100–300 mg/kg IV of 10% calcium gluconate solution. Hyponatremia ($\leq$125 mg/dL) should be corrected with 3% saline, 5 to 10 mL/kg IV [4].

Box 2. Causes of seizures in infants

First day of life

    Anoxia/hypoxia
    Drugs
    Hypoglycemia/hyperglycemia
    Infection
    Intracranial hemorrhage
    Pyridoxine deficiency
    Trauma

Second day of life

    Benign familial neonatal seizures
    Congenital anomalies or developmental brain disorders
    Drug withdrawal
    Hyperphosphatemia
    Hypertension
    Hypocalcemia
    Hypoglycemia
    Hyponatremia/hypernatremia
    Inborn errors of metabolism
    Sepsis
    Trauma

Day 4 to 6 months of age

    Benign idiopathic neonatal seizures
    Congenital anomalies or developmental brain disorders
    Drug withdrawal
    Hyperphosphatemia
    Hypertension
    Hypocalcemia
    Hyponatremia/hypernatremia
    Inborn errors of metabolism
    Infection

After the seizure has stopped, a CT scan or ultrasonogram of the head should be obtained, and a sepsis evaluation should be completed. Broad-spectrum antibiotics should be administered, and the initiation of antiviral therapy (acyclovir) should be considered. The treatment for sepsis or meningitis should not be delayed if a lumbar puncture cannot be performed at the time. All neonates

Table 1
Pharmaceutical management of neonatal seizures

Drug	Dosage
Benzodiazepines	
Lorazepam	0.05–0.1 mg/kg IV
Diazepam	0.2–0.3 mg/kg IV or 0.5 mg/kg rectal
Midazolam	0.1 mg/kg IV or 0.2 mg/kg intramuscular
Phenobarbital	20 mg/kg IV initially then repeat 10 mg/kg IV q10 min (maximum of 50–60 mg/kg)
Phenytoin/fosphenytoin	15–20 mg/kg IV

with seizures require admission to the hospital for observation and completion of the evaluation.

Nonaccidental head trauma: shaken baby syndrome

The terms nonaccidental head trauma or shaken baby syndrome (SBS) are more recent terms that were adapted from Caffee's [6] landmark 1974 article, which introduced the concept of "the whiplash shaken baby syndrome." The diagnosis of nonaccidental trauma may be challenging, depending on the presenting signs and symptoms. In fact, one study found that 31% of infants with unrecognized abuse had been evaluated previously by a physician [7]. Nonaccidental trauma is an important diagnosis to consider in an infant with a suspicious history or nonspecific symptoms because the long-term morbidity from SBS is as high as 70%, and mortality is as high as 30% [8,9]. Although these infants may have no external signs of trauma, the presence of any scalp hematoma is associated with an increased incidence of intracranial hemorrhage.

The initial management should include ABC stabilization as well as a thorough physical examination that includes an attempt to visualize the retinas for hemorrhages. While obtaining IV access, blood may be obtained for a complete blood count, platelet count, prothrombin time, and partial thromboplastin time. Further laboratory evaluation, including cultures and bedside glucose evaluation, will be determined by the clinical presentation. Once the infant is stabilized, a CT of the head should be performed. These infants should be admitted to the hospital for further medical evaluation, management, and investigation by the appropriate authorities. Any suspicion of nonaccidental trauma should be reported from the emergency department.

Apparent life-threatening event

An apparent life-threatening event (ALTE) is defined as "an episode that is frightening to the observer that is characterized by some combination of apnea, color change, marked change in muscle tone, choking or gagging. In some cases the observer fears that the infant has died" [10]. Because the diagnosis is subjective and dependent on the observer's interpretation, the ED evaluation will

---

Box 3. Common differential diagnosis of an apparent life-threatening event

Acid-base disturbance
Anemia
Botulism
Child abuse
Dysrhythmias
Electrolyte abnormalities
Gastroesophageal reflux
Hypoglycemia
Hypothermia seizures
Inborn errors of metabolism
Intracranial hemorrhage
Meningitis and encephalitis
Pertussis
Pneumonia
RSV
Sepsis

---

vary depending on the available history and physical examination of the neonate. One study found that only 2.5% of patients presenting with an ALTE had positive diagnostic tests [11]. Box 3 provides a list of the more common causes of an ALTE. The workup may include a full sepsis evaluation, electrolytes, chest radiography (CXR), ECG, and respiratory syncytial virus (RSV) and pertussis nasal swabs. Hospitalization for observation and monitoring is appropriate.

Respiratory emergencies: bronchiolitis

Although respiratory distress in a neonate is usually obvious, finding the underlying cause may be more challenging. Respiratory symptoms are most commonly a result of pulmonary problems but may be also caused by cardiac, central nervous system, metabolic, endocrine, or gastrointestinal (GI) emergencies. Lower airway abnormalities such as congenital pulmonary malformations, including a diaphragmatic hernia, tracheoesophageal fistula, cystic adenomatous malformation, and congenital lobar emphysema, and upper airway lesions such as laryngo- or tracheomalacia or airway hemangioma may be the reason for the respiratory distress. Because respiratory failure is the most common cause of cardiac arrest in children, aggressive and early interventions may be life saving.

Bronchiolitis is the most common cause of respiratory disease in children less than 2 years of age [12]. The respiratory syncytial virus is responsible 80% of the time, but other viral causes include the adenovirus, influenza, and parainfluenza viruses [12]. Epidemics occur usually in the winter and spring months. Presenting symptoms include nasal congestion, tachypnea, wheezing, retractions, and apnea. Apnea may be an early symptom, appearing before any respiratory symptoms have developed.

ED management includes ABC stabilization and an initial CXR. Other diagnostic interventions will be directed by the clinical presentation. Pharmacologic treatment may include a trial of nebulized epinephrine or a β-agonist. Epinephrine may be beneficial in initially improving respiratory distress but has not been shown to significantly shorten the length of stay compared with albuterol [13]. Controversy exists over the use of steroids in children with bronchiolitis. However, although corticosteroids have not been demonstrated to have significant benefit in the management of either mild or severe bronchiolitis [14], there may be a subset of patients who do respond to steroid use. Patients with recurrent episodes of wheezing, a strong family history of atopy, or severe disease on presentation may be candidates for therapy. The overall mortality of previously healthy infants hospitalized with RSV is ≤1%, but those infants who are at high risk (eg, have an underlying disease such as coronary heart disease, chronic lung disease, or prematurity) have an overall mortality of 3.5% [15].

Neonates with bronchiolitis who demonstrate any respiratory distress or apnea should be admitted to a monitored bed for supportive care. In addition, special consideration should be given to infants with comorbid conditions.

Infectious emergencies

As with other neonatal emergencies, the presenting signs and symptoms may range from minor complaints to shock. Fever (≥100.4°F, rectally) should always prompt a full evaluation for sepsis, but other symptoms, including hypothermia and irritability, may be just as concerning. An undeveloped immune system and recent exposure to bacteria present in the birth canal put the neonate at high risk for developing a severe bacterial illness. These infections include sepsis, meningitis, skin infections, pneumonia, and osteomyelitis. A pertinent birth history should include maternal group B streptococcal status, the presence of a sexually transmitted disease, prolonged rupture of membranes, mode of delivery, and any invasive monitoring (eg, a scalp monitor) should increase suspicion for a severe bacterial illness.

Sepsis

A full sepsis evaluation should be initiated in any neonate with a fever or other nonspecific symptoms that do not have an obvious explanation. In fact, finding a possible source (including RSV) should not limit the evaluation. Each sepsis evaluation should include a CBC, blood culture, urinalysis, urine culture (catheterized or suprapubic specimen), CXR, and lumbar puncture for the analysis of cerebrospinal fluid (CSF). In addition, broad-spectrum antibiotics (Table 2)

Table 2
Recommended antibiotics and dosages for neonatal sepsis

Antibiotic	Dosage
Ampicillin	50–100 mg/kg IV
Gentamycin	2 mg/kg IV
Cefotaxime	50–100 mg/kg IV
Acylovir	20 mg/kg IV

should be administered, and the neonate should be admitted to the hospital, regardless of normal laboratory and radiographic findings.

Neonatal herpes

Neonatal herpes is an uncommon diagnosis but has an increasing incidence, with a rate of 2000 neonatal infections per year in the United States [16]. The symptoms may be subtle, without skin findings, but should not be excluded because 17% to 39% of cases never have skin lesions [17]. A high index of suspicion is important because early detection and treatment with acyclovir, 20 mg/kg IV, has been shown to decrease the mortality from 90% to 31% [18]. Despite this improvement, the long-term morbidity remains high. Treatment should be considered in any patient with fever, irritability, abnormal CSF findings, and especially seizures. Laboratory evaluation should include an analysis of a CSF biopsy for herpes simplex virus by polymerase chain reaction, viral culture, and liver function tests. A CXR may demonstrate pneumonitis. Management should include supportive care, broad-spectrum antibiotics for sepsis, and administration of acyclovir. Critically ill neonates or those with a high suspicion for neonatal herpes should be admitted to a monitored bed and receive critical care support.

Dermatologic infections

Neonatal skin infections deserve special mention because a full sepsis evaluation is warranted. The antibiotic coverage should be expanded to include an anti-staphylococcal agent. Nafcillin, 50 mg/kg IV, may be appropriate, but the use of this drug should be determined by the resistance profile in the community.

Omphalitis, an umbilical and periumbilical infection, is considered a surgical emergency if it extends to the peritoneum, and it requires ABC stabilization, fluid resuscitation, IV antibiotics (ampicillin, gentamicin, and flagyl), and immediate pediatric surgical consultation. Any erythema that surrounds the umbilicus and extends to the abdominal wall is suspicious for omphalitis, regardless of the presence of fever, and the infant should undergo a septic evaluation, the initiation of antibiotics, and hospital admission.

Gastrointestinal emergencies

Although acute viral gastroenteritis may present in the neonatal period and should be evaluated with specific concern for hydration status, the life-threatening diseases should always be excluded first. Symptoms of GI emergencies may be subtle, including irritability or feeding intolerance, or they may be more apparent, with vomiting (bilious or nonbilious), abdominal distention, and shock. GI emergencies are discussed more extensively elsewhere in this issue.

Malrotation with midgut volvulus

Any history of bilious emesis should be considered midgut volvulus until it is proven otherwise. Malrotation occurs in 1 in 5000 live births, and approximately 80% of cases present with volvulus in the first month of life [19]. The initial evaluation should include ABC stabilization, fluid resuscitation, nasogastric tube placement, and abdominal radiographs. The most common radiographic finding in the case of malrotation with volvulus is a normal gas pattern [20]. With severe duodenal obstruction, a "double bubble sign" may be present. An upper GI is the study of choice for definitive diagnosis. Immediate pediatric surgical consultation is imperative.

Necrotizing enterocolitis

Necrotizing enterocolitis (NEC) is, classically, a disease of premature neonates but may also present in the term infant. Symptoms may include feeding difficulties, irritability, abdominal distention, and hematochezia. Management includes ABC stabilization, fluid resuscitation, and the administration of antibiotics. Laboratory evaluation should include a CBC, blood culture, and serum electrolytes. The classic radiographic finding is pneumatosis intestinalis or portal air. Free air may be present if the bowel has already perforated. Management should include surgical consultation and admission to a critical care service.

Toxic megacolon

Hirshsprung's disease occurs in 1 in 5000 live births, with a male:female ratio of 4:1 [21]. This condition results from the failure of neural crest cells to migrate in the colon, resulting in an aganglionic section of bowel. This diagnosis should be considered in the presence of constipation or failure to pass meconium in the first 24 hours of life.

Enterocolitis (toxic megacolon) may develop in these patients and may present similarly to NEC. The management and stabilization are also similar. A radiograph may demonstrate an enlarged or dilated section of colon. These patients also warrant a surgical consultation and should receive critical care management.

Table 3
Management of hyperbilirubinemia in newborns

	Total serum bilirubin (mg/dL)				
	Postnatal time				
Risk category	24 h day 1	36 h day 1.5	48 h day 2	72 h day 3	96 h day 4
High risk (35–37 wks gestational age + risk factors)	8	9	11	13	14
Medium risk (≥38 wks gestational age + risk factors, or 35–37 wks and well)	10	12	13	15	17
For photo-therapy in infants ≥ 35 weeks' gestation					
Total bilirubin value is used					
Risk factors include: isoimmune hemolytic disease, asphyxia, G6PD deficiency, sepsis, acidosis, lethargy, temperature instability, or albumin < 3.0 g/dL					
Guidelines are for phototherapy use, which is indicated when total serum bilirubin values exceed those values within the table					

Data from the American Academy of Pediatrics Clinical Practice Guidelines (Subcommittee on Hyperbilirubinemia. Management of hyperbilirubinemia in the newborn infant 35 or more weeks of gestation. Pediatrics 2004;114:297–307.

Hyperbilirubinemia

Neonatal hyperbilirubinemia (jaundice) is a common newborn finding that, although usually is benign, may represent a more serious underlying diagnosis. The level of concern will be directed by the age of presentation, associated clinical symptoms, and most importantly, if the bilirubin is primarily unconjugated (indirect) or there is an elevated conjugated (direct) portion. As a result, the initial evaluation should include a total and direct bilirubin test, hematocrit level, reticulocyte count, and Coombs' test. The causes of unconjugated hyperbilirubinemia are usually physiologic or related to breast feeding but may also include ABO or other minor blood group incompatibilities, spherocytosis, glucose-6-phosphate dehydrogenase deficiency, sepsis, Gilbert's disease, or Crigler-Najjar syndrome. Conjugated hyperbilirubinemia is always a condition

Table 4
American Academy of Pediatrics recommendations for phototherapy and exchange transfusion in the healthy term (≥ 38 wk) neonate

Age (h)	Phototherapy (g/dL)	Exchange (g/dL)
24	12	19
48	15	22
72	18	24
≥ 96	20	25

Data from Colletti JE, Homme JL, Woodridge DP. Unsuspected neonatal killers in emergency medicine. Emerg Med Clin North Am 2004;22:929–60.

Presence of ill-appearing infant, unstable vital signs, lethargy, apnea, tachypnea, fever, poor feeding, or behavior change

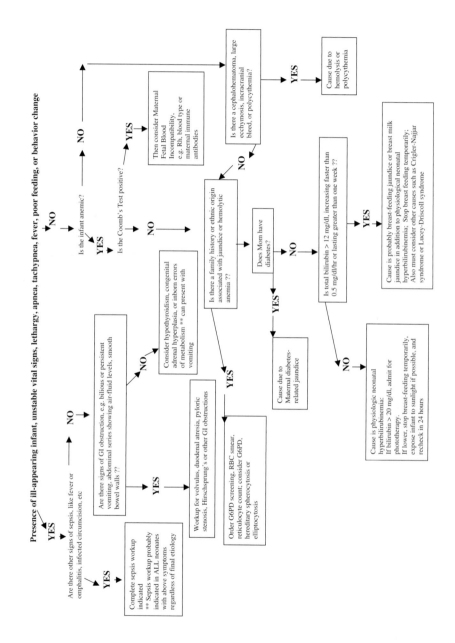

Box 4. Presenting signs and symptoms of an inborn error of metabolism

Subtle

    Abnormal Tone
    Irritability
    Poor feeding or feeding refusal
    Poor weight gain
    Somnolence
    Tachycardia
    Tachypnea
    Vomiting

Overt

    Acidosis
    Altered thermoregulation
    Apnea
    Arrhythmia
    Cardiomyopathy
    Dehydration
    Lethargy or Coma
    Persistent hypoglycemia
    Poor perfusion or hypotension
    Seizures
    Sudden unexplained death

---

of concern, and the differential diagnosis includes biliary atresia or obstruction, hepatitis, and α_1-antitrypsin deficiency. The current management criteria for unconjugated hyperbilirubinemia are outlined in Tables 3 and 4. Fig. 1 shows an algorithm for the evaluation of these neonates. Hospitalization and further evaluation of infants with conjugated hyperbilirubinemia typically is warranted.

Metabolic emergencies: inborn errors of metabolism

Inborn errors of metabolism (IEM) are uncommon but remain a source of anxiety in considering the diagnosis. Each state screens for specific defects of

---

Fig. 1. Inborn errors of metabolism. Exceptions have been noted to the pathway as shown. (Courtesy of Ken Kwon, MD, University of California, Irvine, CA).

metabolism, and the only consistency from state to state is screening for phenyl-ketonuria, congenital hypothyroidism, and galactosemia [22]. A high index of suspicion is important because the symptoms may be subtle, and early recognition and interventions may significantly affect long-term morbidity. Box 4 summarizes the subtle and overt symptoms that may suggest an IEM.

The initial ED management should include ABC stabilization and a bedside blood glucose test. Laboratory evaluation should include serum electrolytes, pH level, lactate, ammonia, CBC, liver function tests and urinalysis for reducing substances, and ketones. The presence of ketones in the neonate's urine should increase suspicion for an IEM because the errors are typically inefficient producers of ketones even in the presence of hypoglycemia [23]. Other diagnostic tests should include blood and urine for amino and organic acids. The presence or absence of hyperammonemia and pH level are helpful diagnostically in differentiating between several defects. Fig. 2 provides a diagnostic pathway for normal and elevated serum ammonia. The correction of electrolytes (specifically providing parenteral glucose to prevent catabolism), fluid resuscitation, admission to the hospital for further evaluation, discontinuation of all feedings, and consultation with a pediatric geneticist are all important steps in the initial management of an IEM.

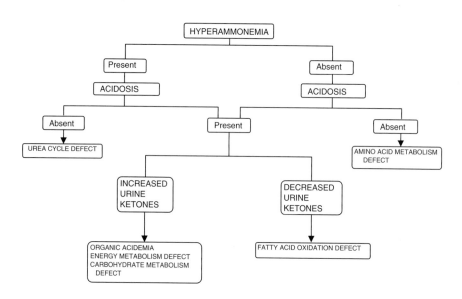

Note: exceptions to above pathway exist.
Courtesy of Ken Kwon,MD. University of California, Irvine

Fig. 2. Management of neonatal jaundice caused by unconjugated bilirubin. (Courtesy of Maureen McCollough, MD, Keck USC School of Medicine, Pasadena, CA).

Endocrine emergencies

Congenital adrenal hyperplasia

The most common cause of congenital adrenal hyperplasia (CAH) is the result of a deficiency in the 21-hydroxylase enzyme [24]. There is no routine screening in all states for this defect, and male neonates may not have any physical genitalia abnormalities that are noticed in the newborn nursery. As a result, these infants with an unrecognized diagnosis of CAH may present to the ED with shock during the first 2 weeks of life. An initial evaluation that reveals hyponatremia, hyperkalemia, and hypotension unresponsive to fluids or inotropes should immediately prompt the consideration of CAH. Hypoglycemia is also a common finding. Management other than ABC stabilization should include replacement of steroids with hydrocortisone, 25 to 50 mg/m^2 IV [4]. The infant with CAH has a deficiency of steroids, which disables a normal stress response. These infants should be admitted to an appropriate facility that provides pediatric subspecialty and critical care support.

Thyrotoxicosis

Infants born to mothers with Graves' disease may develop thyrotoxicosis and present with delayed symptoms to the ED. Symptoms at presentation may include poor feeding, irritability, tachycardia, respiratory distress, hyperthermia, or congestive heart failure. In the presence of these symptoms, laboratory evaluation should include thyroid functions tests. Treatment may require propranolol, 0.25 mg/kg IV, to control tachycardia. In addition, propylthiouracil, 1.25 mg/kg IV, followed by Lugol's solution (1–5 drops orally) should be administered to help control the hypermetabolic state and hormone release [24]. These patients, once stabilized, should be admitted to a pediatric subspecialty hospital.

Cardiac disease

Acyanotic heart disease

Clinical decompensation in acyanotic heart diseases may be a result of closure of the ductus arteriosus (DA). The onset of symptoms typically is gradual, with the onset of congestive heart failure. Different degrees of obstruction to the left ventricular outflow tract are present that result in an increase in pulmonary blood flow and a gradual development of heart failure. The classic triad of symptoms for pediatric congestive heart failure is tachypnea, tachycardia, and hepatomegaly. In addition, there may be a history of poor feeding, sweating or color change with feedings, and poor weight gain. Lower extremity edema and jugular venous distention are unlikely findings at this age. The more common causes of acyanotic heart disease are listed in Box 5 [25].

Box 5. Causes of acyanotic heart disease that present with congestive heart failure

Anemia
Aortic atresia
Aortic stenosis
Arteriovenous malformation
Coarctation of the Aorta
Complete arteriovenous canal
Cor pulmonale caused by bronchopulmonary dysplasia
Endocardial cushion defect
Hypoplastic left heart
Interrupted aortic arch
Mitral valve atresia
Patent ductus arteriosus
Truncus arteriosus
Ventricular septal defect

The evaluation should include a CXR, ECG, and serum electrolytes. The initial management may also be administration of prostaglandin E (PGE)$_1$, but success is less likely because the development of heart failure is gradual and the DA may already have been closed for several days to weeks. The first-line choice in pharmacologic management of congestive heart failure is furosemide, 1 mg/kg IV; however, other adjuvants include dopamine, dobutamine, and digoxin. Pediatric cardiology consultation should be obtained, and once stabilized, the patient should be transported to the appropriate facility.

Cyanotic heart disease

Cyanotic congenital heart defects that are not detected in the newborn nursery will present during the first 2 to 3 weeks of life when the DA closes. With the

---

Box 6. Causes of cyanotic heart disease: the five "terrible Ts" (and one "S")

1. Transposition of the great vessels
2. Total anomalous pulmonary venous return
3. Tetralogy of Fallot
4. Truncus arteriosus
5. Tricuspid atresia
6. Severe pulmonic stenosis

---

neonate's first breath, oxygen and other mediators stimulate the closure of the DA. Functional closure of the ductus occurs in the first 10 to 14 hours of life, but anatomic closure may not occur until 2 to 3 weeks of age because of prematurity, acidosis, and hypoxia [26]. The congenital heart defects that classically present with cyanosis, commonly referred to as the "terrible Ts," are listed in Box 6.

The immediate goal in evaluating a cyanotic neonate is to differentiate between cardiac and noncardiac causes. The classic hyperoxia test is carried out by obtaining an arterial blood gas (ABG), then placing the patient on 100% oxygen for 10 minutes and then by repeating the ABG. If the cause of cyanosis is pulmonary, the PaO_2 should increase by 30 mm Hg, but if the cause is cardiac, there should be minimal improvement in the PaO_2. The initial ABG should be obtained with co-oximetry because methemoglobinemia may also cause cyanosis in the neonatal period. A simpler method for completing the hyperoxia test is to provide 100% oxygen and observe the oxygen saturation on pulse oximetry for an increase of 10% in pulmonary causes and minimal change with cyanotic heart disease. A CXR and ECG should also be obtained, but these modalities usually are not specific for the diagnosis of congenital heart disease. Although it is not routinely available in the ED, an echocardiogram is diagnostic.

If the neonate's oxygen saturation or PaO_2 fail to improve and cyanotic heart disease is suspected, then PGE_1 should be administered as a bolus of 0.05 µg/kg IV followed by an infusion of 0.05 to 0.1 µg/kg /min IV [4]. Age-appropriate airway equipment should be immediately available before starting PGE_1 because a non-dose-dependent side effect of PGE_1 is apnea, which requires intubation and mechanical ventilation. It may take 10 to 15 minutes for a response to PGE_1, and its effect can be recognized by an increase in oxygen saturation. The patient should be weaned from supplemental oxygen as soon as possible after the oxygen saturation has improved. After stabilization, the patient should be transported to an appropriate facility for pediatric cardiology and pediatric cardiovascular surgery consultation.

Summary

The differential diagnosis for each subtle or nonspecific symptom in the neonatal evaluation is extensive. This review categorizes the more common life-threatening illnesses by system, in an attempt to provide a guide to the initial recognition, evaluation, and emergency department management. It is important to keep a high index of suspicion when evaluating the neonate because some initial interventions may be life saving.

References

[1] Nordli DR, Bazil CW, Scheuer NIL, et al. Recognition and classification of seizures in infants. Epilepsia 1997;38:553–60.

[2] Mizrahi EM, Kellaway P. Characterization and classification of neonatal seizures. Neurology 1987;37:1837–44.

[3] Volpe JJ. Neonatal seizures: current concepts and revised classification. Pediatrics 1989;84: 422–8.

[4] Gunn VL, Nechyba C, editors. The Harriet Lane handbook. 16th edition. St. Louis (MO): Mosby; 2002.

[5] Maytal J, Novak GP, King KC. Lorazepam in the treatment of refractory seizures. J Child Neurol 1991;6:319–23.

[6] Caffee J. The whiplash shaken infant syndrome: manual shaking by the extremities with whiplash-induced intracranial and intraocular bleedings, linked with residual permanent brain damage and mental retardation. Pediatrics 1974;54:369–403.

[7] Jenny C, Hymel KP, Ritzen A, et al. Analysis of missed cases of abusive head trauma. JAMA 1999;281(7):621–6.

[8] Jayawant S, Rawlinson A, Gibbon F, et al. Subdural haemorrhages in infants: population based study. BMJ 1998;317:1558–61.

[9] Haviland J, Russell RI. Outcome after severe non-accidental head injury. Arch Dis Child 1997; 77(6):504–7.

[10] Little GA, Ballard RA, Brooks JG, et al. National Institute of Health consensus development: course on infantile apnea and home monitoring, September 1986. Pediatrics 1987;79:292–9.

[11] DePiero AD, Teach SJ, Chamberlain JM. ED evaluation of infants after an apparent life-threatening event. Am J Emerg Med 2004;22:83–6.

[12] Law BJ, De Carvalho V, for the Pediatric Investigators Collaborative Network on Infections in Canada. Respiratory syncytial virus infections in hospitalized Canadian children: regional differences in patient populations and management practices. Pediatr Infect Dis J 1993;12:659–63.

[13] Wainwright C, Altamirano L, Cheney J, et al. A multicenter, randomized, double-blind, controlled trial of nebulized epinephrine in infants with acute bronchiolitis. N Engl J Med 2003; 349:27–35.

[14] Garrison MM, Christakis DA, Harvey E, et al. Systemic corticosteroids in infant bronchiolitis: a meta-analysis. An Pediatr (Barc) 2000;105(4):e4.

[15] Navas L, Wang E, De Carvalho V, et al for the Pediatric Investigators Collaborative Network on Infections in Canada. Improved outcome of respiratory syncytial virus infection in a high-risk hospitalized population of Canadian children. J Pediatr 1992;121:348–54.

[16] Enright AM, Prober CG. Neonatal herpes infection: diagnosis, treatment, and prevention. Semin Neonatol 2002;7:283–91.

[17] Kimberlin DW, Lin CY, Jacobs RF, et al. Natural history of neonatal herpes simplex virus infections in the acyclovir era. Pediatrics 2001;108:223–9.

[18] Kimberlin DW, Lin CY, Jacobs RF, et al. Safety and efficacy of high dose intravenous acyclovir in the management of neonatal herpes simplex virus infections. Pediatric 2001;108:230–8.

[19] Irish MS, Pearl RH, Caty MG, et al. The approach to common abdominal diagnosis in infants and children. Pediatr Clin North Am 1998;45(4):729–72.

[20] Berdon WE, Baker DH, Bull S, et al. Midgut malrotation and volvulus: which films are most helpful? Radiology 1970;96:375–83.

[21] Swenson O. Hirshprung disease. Pediatr Rev 2002;109(5):914–7.

[22] Newborn screening: characteristics of state programs. GAO-03-449; 2003.

[23] Chakrapani A, Cleary MA, Wraith JE. Detection of inborn errors of metabolism in the newborn. Arch Dis Child Fetal Neonatal Ed 2001;84:F205–10.

[24] Kabbani MD. Congenital adrenal hyperplasia: epidemiology, management and practical drug treatment. Pediatr Drugs 2001;3(8):599–611.

[25] Brousseau T, Sharieff GQ. Improving neonatal emergency care: critical concepts. Pediatric Emergency Medicine Reports 2005;10:49–60.

[26] Hammerman C. Patent ductus arteriosus: clinical relevance of prostaglandins and prostaglandin inhibitors in PDA pathophysiology and treatment. Clin Perinatol 1995;22(2):457–79.

ELSEVIER
SAUNDERS

Pediatr Clin N Am 53 (2006) 85–105

PEDIATRIC CLINICS

OF NORTH AMERICA

Pediatric Dysrhythmias

Stephanie J. Doniger, MD, FAAP*,
Ghazala Q. Sharieff, MD, FACEP, FAAEM, FAAP

Pediatric Emergency Medicine, Children's Hospital and Health Center/
University of California San Diego, 3020 Children's Way, MC 5075 San Diego, CA 92123-4282, USA

The overall incidence of arrhythmias is 13.9 per 100,000 emergency department (ED) visits and 55.1 per 100,000 pediatric ED visits (children under 18 years of age) [1]. Among children with arrhythmias, the most common dysrhythmias are sinus tachycardia (50%), supraventricular tachycardia (13%), bradycardia (6%), and atrial fibrillation (4.6%) [1].

The presentation of dysrhythmias can serve as a diagnostic challenge to most clinicians because most children present with vague and nonspecific symptoms such as "fussiness" or "difficulty feeding." Despite the infrequency and vague presenting symptoms, it is critical to identify and appropriately manage these disorders. When left they are unrecognized and untreated, dysrhythmias can lead to cardiopulmonary compromise and arrest.

The electrocardiogram in pediatrics

The most common reasons for obtaining EKGs in children are chest pain, suspected dysrhythmias, seizures, syncope, drug exposure, electrical burns, electrolyte abnormalities, and abnormal physical examination findings. Of all of these, the most life-threatening findings are those caused by electrolyte disturbances, drug exposure, and burns [2].

Although a complete EKG interpretation is beyond the scope of this chapter, it is advisable to use a systematic approach, with special attention to rate, rhythm, axis, ventricular and atrial hypertrophy, and the presence of any ischemia or

---

* Corresponding author.
E-mail address: sdoniger@sbcglobal.net (S.J. Doniger).

Table 1
Pediatric ECG normal intervals

Age	Heart rate (BPM)	PR interval (s)	QRS interval (s)
1st wk	90–160	0.08–0.15	0.03–0.08
1–3wk	100–180	0.08–0.15	0.03–0.08
1–2 mo	120–180	0.08–0.15	0.03–0.08
3–5 mo	105–185	0.08–0.15	0.03–0.08
6–11 mo	110–170	0.07–0.16	0.03–0.08
1–2 y	90–165	0.08–0.16	0.03–0.08
3–4 y	70–140	0.09–0.17	0.04–0.08
5–7 y	65–140	0.09–0.17	0.04–0.08
8–11 y	60–130	0.09–0.17	0.04–0.09
12–15 y	65–130	0.09–0.18	0.04–0.09
≥16 y	50–120	0.12–0.20	0.05–0.10

Courtesy of Ra'id Abdullah, MD, University of Chicago, IL.

repolarization abnormalities. More specifically, it is essential to interpret pediatric EKG's based on age-specific rates and intervals (Table 1) [3–5]. The EKG can be evaluated further for rhythm, chamber size, and T-wave morphology.

Tachydysrhythmias

Tachycardia is defined as a heart rate beyond the upper limit of normal for the patient's age. In adults, the heart rate is greater than 100 beats per minute (BPM). Tachycardias can be classified broadly into those that originate from loci above the atrioventricular (AV) node (ie, supraventricular), from the AV node (AV node reentrant tachycardias), and from the ventricle. The majority of tachycardias are supraventricular (SVT) in origin. Those that are ventricular in origin are associated typically with hemodynamic compromise [4]. When tachycardia is recognized, step-wise questioning can help evaluate the EKG tracing. Is it regular or irregular? Is the QRS complex narrow or wide? Does every P wave result in a single QRS complex? Once these have been established, the treatment options are considered according to whether the patient has a pulse and the presenting rhythm on EKG (Fig. 1) [6].

Sinus tachycardia

Sinus tachycardia can be differentiated from other tachycardias by a narrow QRS axis and a P wave that precedes every QRS complex. The rate is usually greater than 140 BPM in children and greater than 160 BPM in infants. Sinus tachycardia is typically benign. The pulse rate has been shown to increase linearly with temperature in children older than 2 months of age. For every 1°C (1.8°F) increase in body temperature, the pulse rate increases by an average of 9.6 BPM [7]. Sinus tachycardia can also be associated with such underlying conditions as

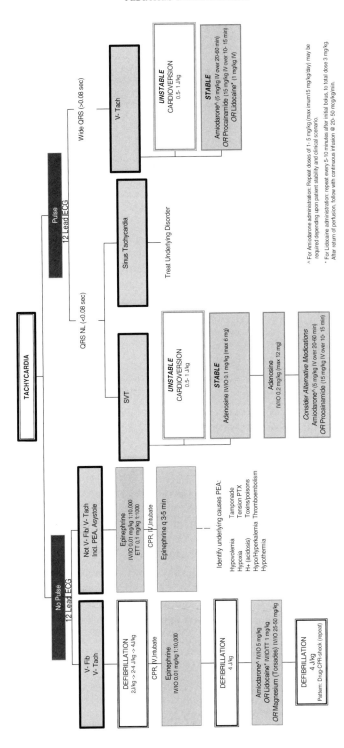

Fig. 1. Tachycardia algorithm. PEA, pulseless electrical activity; SVT, supraventricular tachycardia; V-Fib, ventricular fibrillation; V-Tach, ventricular tachycardia. (*Data from* Hazinski M, Zaritsky A, Nadkarini V, et al. PALS provider manual. Dallas (TX): American Heart Association; 2002.)

hypoxia, anemia, hypovolemia, shock, myocardial ischemia, pulmonary edema, hyperthyroidism, medications (catecholamines), hypocalcemia, and illicit drug use. Most commonly, it is a result of dehydration and hypovolemia [1,4]. Because children augment cardiac output by increasing the heart rate rather than the stroke volume, heart rate increases appear early, whereas hypotension is a late sign of dehydration. Treatment aimed at correcting the heart rate alone may be harmful to the patient because the tachycardia is a compensatory response to sustain adequate cardiac output. For this reason, the treatment of sinus tachycardia is largely targeted at treating the underlying disorder, rather than treating the tachycardia itself.

Ventricular tachycardia

Although it is rare in children, ventricular tachycardia is an important rhythm to recognize and treat promptly. Nonperfusing ventricular rhythms are seen in up to 19% of pediatric cardiac arrests, when sudden infant death syndrome (SIDS) cases are excluded [8]. Although the heart may be contracting and pulses are palpable in some patients who have ventricular tachycardia, those contractions are hemodynamically inefficient and can lead ultimately to syncope and death if left untreated. Furthermore, ventricular tachycardia can decompensate into ventricular fibrillation, which is a nonperfusing, terminal arrhythmia.

Ventricular tachycardia may result from electrolyte disturbances (hyperkalemia, hypokalemia, and hypocalcemia), metabolic abnormalities, congenital heart disorders, myocarditis, or drug toxicity. Other causes include cardiomyopathies, cardiac tumors, acquired heart disease, prolonged QT syndrome, and idiopathic causes.

On electrocardiograms, the QRS complexes have a wide configuration. The QRS duration is prolonged, ranging from 0.06 to 0.14 seconds. Complexes may appear monomorphic with a uniform contour and absent or retrograde P waves. Alternatively, the QRS complexes may appear polymorphic or vary randomly as is seen in torsades de pointes. EKG findings that further support the presence of ventricular tachycardia include the presence of AV dissociation with the ventricular rate exceeding the atrial rate (Fig. 2).

In a patient who has ventricular tachycardia, the urgency of treatment depends on the patient's clinical status. Initially, the airway, breathing, and circulation (ABCs) must be maintained, and it must be determined whether the patient has a pulse and is hemodynamically stable. The American Heart Association has set forth treatment algorithms [6] to facilitate prompt treatment for this potentially fatal rhythm (see Fig. 1).

Ventricular tachycardia with a pulse in an unstable patient warrants immediate synchronized cardioversion at 0.5 to 1 J/kg. It is important to pretreat conscious patients with light sedation (eg, midazolam, 0.1 mg/kg). Pharmacologic interventions include amiodarone (5 mg/kg intravenously [IV] over 20–60 min; maximum single dose, 150 mg; maximum daily dose, 15 mg/kg/d), procainamide (15 mg IV over 30–60 min), or lidocaine (1 mg/kg IV bolus, repeat every

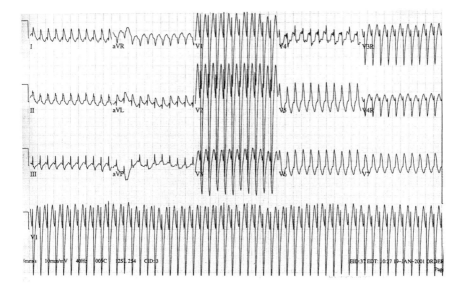

Fig. 2. Ventricular tachycardia. An example of an extraordinarily fast ventricular tachycardia, with a heart rate of almost 300 BPM. (Courtesy of CDR Jonathan T. Fleenor, MD, Naval Medical Center, San Diego, CA.)

5–10 min, with max total of 3 mg/kg) [9]. When using procainamide, the infusion is stopped once the arrhythmia resolves if the QRS complex widens to ≥50% over the baseline or if hypotension ensues. Pulseless ventricular tachycardia should be treated as ventricular fibrillation (see below).

After cardioversion, the return to normal sinus rhythm is usually transient. The medication used to achieve sinus rhythm must be given as a continuous infusion using lidocaine (20–50 µg/kg/min), amiodarone (7–15 mg/kg/d), or procainamide (20–80 µg/kg/min [maximum dose of 2 g/24 h]) [6]. In polymorphic ventricular tachycardia, temporary atrial or ventricular pacing may be required. Overall, the treatment goal is to keep the heart rate at less than 150 BPM in infants and less than 130 BPM in older children.

Premature ventricular contractions

A premature ventricular contraction (PVC) is a premature, wide QRS complex that has a distinct configuration and is not preceded by a P wave. They may appear in a pattern of two consecutive PVCs (couplet), an alternating PVC with a normal QRS complex (bigeminy), or in which every third beat is a PVC (trigeminy). The occurrence of three or more consecutive PVCs is considered ventricular tachycardia. The sinoatrial (SA) node maintains a normal conduction pace, and the PVC replaces a normal QRS wave while maintaining a rhythm.

Although most children who have PVCs are otherwise healthy, PVCs can also be associated with congenital heart disease, mitral valve prolapse, prolonged QT syndrome, and cardiomyopathies (dilated and hypertrophic). Malignant origins include electrolyte imbalances, drug toxicities (eg, general anesthesia, digoxin, catecholamines, amphetamines, sympathomimetics, and phenothiazines), cardiac injury, cardiac tumors, myocarditis (Lyme and viral diseases), hypoxia, and an intraventricular catheter.

For the most part, patients who have PVCs are asymptomatic; however, when they are unrecognized and untreated, there is a risk of developing ventricular tachycardia in patients who have a serious underlying cause. When they are examined, 50% to 75% of otherwise normal children may have PVCs seen on Holter monitoring [4]. It is crucial to determine whether the heart has an underlying pathology. This can be accomplished by history and physical examination, a 12-lead electrocardiogram, and a chest radiograph. If the findings of all of these tests are normal, no further investigation is necessary.

Premature ventricular contractions are considered malignant if they are associated with underlying heart disease; there is a history of syncope or family history of sudden death; precipitated by or increased with activity; exhibit multiform morphology; they are symptomatic of runs of PVCs; or there are frequent episodes of paroxysmal ventricular tachycardia. Children presenting with premature ventricular contractions require evaluation and possibly treatment in conditions that are likely to cause cardiopulmonary compromise. This occurs whenever there are two or more PVCs in a row, they are multifocal in origin, there is an "R-on-T" phenomenon, or if there is underlying heart disease. The R-on-T phenomenon is an instance in which a PVC occurs on the T wave, which is considered a vulnerable period of stimulating abnormal rhythms. This can be seen with hypoxia or hypokalemia and may result in life-threatening arrhythmias [10]. For those patients who have an underlying cause (eg, electrolyte abnormality, hypoxia, or severe acidosis), the treatment consists of managing the underlying cause. The treatment consists largely of IV lidocaine (1 mg/kg/dose), followed by a lidocaine drip (20–50 µg/kg/min). Amiodarone, procainamide, and β blockers are reserved for conditions that are refractory to lidocaine [11].

In asymptomatic patients who present with isolated PVCs and normal cardiac structure and function, no treatment is necessary. For patients who have couplets, multiform PVS, or frequent PVCs, a referral to a pediatric cardiologist for further investigation is indicated. It is prudent to advise any patient who has PVCs to avoid stimulants such as caffeine, theophylline, and pseudoephedrine because the stimulants may precipitate more frequent PVCs.

Ventricular fibrillation

Ventricular fibrillation is an uncommon rhythm in the pediatric population but is certainly life threatening. The hallmark is chaotic, irregular ventricular contractions without circulation to the body. On the electrocardiogram, the rhythm is one of bizarre QRS complexes with varying sizes and configurations and a rapid, irregular rate. Causes of ventricular fibrillation include postoperative complications from congenital heart disease repair, severe hypoxemia, hyperkalemia, medications (digitalis, quinidine, catecholamines, and anesthesia), myocarditis, and myocardial infarction.

Ventricular fibrillation is an uncommon cause of cardiac arrest in infants less than 1 year of age but increases with growing age. With the increasing use and efficacy of automated external defibrillators (AEDs) in the adult setting, controversy has arisen in the use of AEDs in the prehospital treatment of children in cardiac arrest. Currently, AEDs are approved for patients older than 8 years of age [8]. However, according to the American Heart Association International Liaison Committee on Resuscitation, AEDs may be used in 1- to 8-year-old children who have no signs of circulation, ideally with the pediatric dose. For a lone rescuer responding to a child who does not have signs of circulation, cardiopulmonary resuscitation (CPR) for 1 minute is recommended before attaching an AED or activating emergency medical services. For documented ventricular fibrillation or pulseless ventricular tachycardia, defibrillation is recommended [8].

Because ventricular fibrillation is a nonperfusing rhythm, CPR must be initiated immediately. Of note, ventricular fibrillation is treated the same as ventricular tachycardia without a pulse. Defibrillation is initiated at 2 J/kg, increased from 2 to 4 J/kg, and then followed by a third shock at 4 J/kg. If defibrillation is unsuccessful, epinephrine (0.01 mg/kg, 1:10,000 solution) should be given and repeated every 3 to 5 minutes as necessary.

If pulseless ventricular tachycardia is refractory to defibrillation, antiarrhythmic drugs are indicated, such as amiodarone (5 mg/kg, IV bolus) or lidocaine (1 mg/kg, IV bolus, and repeated to a maximum of 3 mg/kg). Although the pediatric dosing of amiodarone has not been clearly established, the recommended loading dose of 5 mg/kg IV may be given over 20–60 minutes. If rate control is not achieved, the dose may be repeated in increments of 5 mg/kg IV, to a maximum of 15 mg/kg/d IV [12]. For polymorphic ventricular tachycardia (torsades des pointes), the mainstay of treatment is magnesium (20–50 mg/kg, IV).

Supraventricular tachycardia

SVT is the most common symptomatic dysrhythmia in infants and children. In newborns and infants who have SVT, the heart rate is greater than 220 BPM. In older children, it is defined as having a heart rate of more than 180 BPM [13]. The ECG shows a narrow complex tachycardia, either without discernible P waves or with retrograde P waves with an abnormal axis (Fig. 3). The QRS duration is normal but is occasionally increased with aberrancy. It is further characterized by little or no variation in the heart rate.

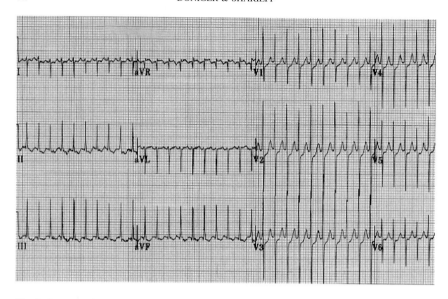

Fig. 3. Supraventricular tachycardia. This 2-week-old infant presented with irritability and emesis. The initial heart rate was in the 300-BPM range, and the infant exhibited grunting and tachypnea. He converted to normal sinus rhythm after the second dose of adenosine was administered. This EKG demonstrates the narrow QRS complexes and the absence of visible P waves. (Courtesy of Stephanie Doniger, MD, Children's Hospital, San Diego, CA.)

There are three types of supraventricular tachycardia. The most common is the AV reentrant tachycardia phenomenon. In addition to the normal conduction from the SA node to the AV node to the bundle of His to the Purkinje fibers, there is an accessory "bypass" pathway in conjunction with the AV node. This pathway is an anatomically separate bypass tract, such as the bundle of Kent, which is seen in Wolff-Parkinson-White (WPW) syndrome. Conduction through this accessory pathway occurs more rapidly than through the normal conduction pathway, creating a cyclic pattern of reentry independent of the SA node. Typical ECG findings of WPW are a short PR interval, a wide QRS, and a positive inflection in the upstroke of the QRS complex, known as the delta wave (Fig. 4). This characteristic finding is evident only after the rhythm is converted to a sinus rhythm [14].

The second type of SVT is the AV nodal, or junctional, tachycardia, which is a cyclical reentrant pattern from dual AV node pathways that are depolarized simultaneously. The third type of SVT, ectopic atrial tachycardia, is rare and is manifested by the rapid firing of a single ectopic focus in the atrium. The hallmark of ectopic atrial tachycardia is the presence of different P-wave morphologies. Each P wave is conducted to the ventricle and, because the ectopic atrial focus is faster than the SA node, it takes over the rate determination [4].

The majority of infants with SVT present at less than 4 months of age, in a male-to-female ratio of 3:2 [15]. Among this group, almost half of the conditions have an idiopathic cause, whereas 24% are associated with conditions such as

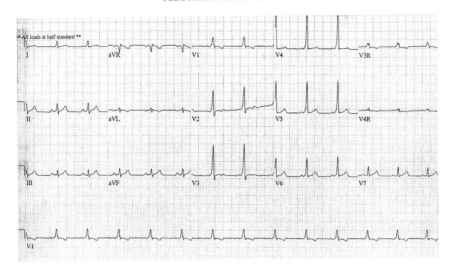

Fig. 4. Wolff-Parkinson-White syndrome. This child presented in supraventricular tachycardia. After being converted to sinus rhythm, the delta waves were apparent. The delta wave is a positive inflection in the upstroke of the QRS complex. (Courtesy of CDR Jonathan T. Fleenor, MD, Naval Medical Center, San Diego, CA.)

fever and drug exposure, 23% are caused by congenital heart disease (most commonly Ebstein's anomaly, single ventricle, L-transposition), and 10% to 20% are the result of WPW syndrome [4]. Among older children, causes are more likely to be WPW, concealed bypass tracts, or congenital heart disease. The AV reentrant type of tachycardia is more common in children less than 12 years of age, whereas the AV node type of tachycardia becomes more evident in adolescents [16]. Other causes include hyperdynamic cardiac activity as is seen in response to catecholamine release, drug use, and postoperative cardiac repair. Toxic causes of SVT include stimulants, β agonists, anticholinergics, salicylates, theophylline, tricyclics, and phenothiazines. Nontoxic causes include anxiety, anemia, sedative and ethanol withdrawal, dehydration, acidosis, exercise, fever, hypoglycemia, hypoxemia, and pain [13].

The diagnosis often begins in triage where the nurse reports a heart rate that is "too fast to count." In newborns and infants who present with SVT, the heart rate is often between 220 and 280 BPM [13]. Most patients do not have an underlying cause to account for the tachycardia, such as fever, dehydration, fluid or blood loss, anxiety, or pain. Infants often present with nonspecific complaints such as "fussiness," lethargy, poor feeding, pallor, sweating with feeds, or simply "not acting right." If congestive heart failure (CHF) is present, caretakers may describe pallor, cough, and respiratory distress. Although many infants can tolerate SVT well for 24 hours, within 48 hours, 50% of them will develop heart failure and may deteriorate rapidly [13]. In contrast, CHF rarely occurs in older children, who are usually able to describe palpitations, chest pain, dizziness, or shortness of breath. Important historical factors include a relationship to exercise, meals, stress, color changes, neurologic changes, or syncope. A medical history significant for cardiac problems, current medications, allergies, or a family history of sudden death or cardiac disease should be investigated.

The management of SVT always begins with ensuring that the patient is maintaining airway, breathing, and cardiovascular status. It is important to promptly administer oxygen and to obtain a 12-lead EKG with a rhythm strip. It is of utmost importance, to expeditiously differentiate between patients who are stable and those who are unstable. In a child presenting with unstable SVT with severe heart failure and poor perfusion, synchronized cardioversion is initiated at 0.5 J/kg and can be increased up to 1 J/kg. Adenosine may be given before cardioversion if intravenous access has already been established. In unstable patients, cardioversion should not be delayed for attempts at IV access or sedation [6].

In children who present with asymptomatic SVT or with mild heart failure, vagal maneuvers such as ice to the face in an infant or blowing through a straw in an older child may be attempted [16]. If that is unsuccessful, adenosine is administered through an IV that is preferably close to the heart. Because of its extremely short half-life, adenosine must be pushed and flushed (with 5 cc normal saline) quickly, to be effective. The initial dose of adenosine is 0.1 mg/kg (up to 6 mg) and can be increased to 0.2 mg/kg/dose (up to 12 mg) if the first dose is ineffective [9]. An effective response is a brief period of asystole on EKG, with the return of a normal sinus rhythm. Failure to terminate the dysrhythmia after the second dose of adenosine in a stable patient should prompt consultation with a pediatric cardiologist. Adenosine can be therapeutic as well as diagnostic; however, it is not effective with nonreciprocating atrial tachycardia, atrial flutter, atrial fibrillation, or ventricular tachycardia. There are minimal hemodynamic consequences associated with adenosine administration [17]. Contraindications include a deinnervated heart (eg, transplant) and second- or third-degree heart block. Additionally, adenosine can worsen bronchospasm in asthmatics and increase heart block or precipitate ventricular arrhythmias in those taking carbamazepine, verapamil, or digoxin.

Alternative medications include procainamide (15 mg/kg, IV, over 30–60 min or at 20–80 μg/kg/min), amiodarone (5 mg/kg over 20–60 min, with a maximum single dose of 150 mg and a maximum daily dose of 15 mg/kg). Of note, amiodarone should not be used in newborns during the first month of life because it contains the preservative benzyl alcohol that has been associated with a gasping syndrome, which is characterized by metabolic acidosis and the "striking onset of gasping respiration, hypotension, bradycardia, and cardiovascular collapse" [18,19]. β blockers such as propranolol or esmolol may be used but with caution because they may induce hypotension [20]. In addition, verapamil should be avoided in children less than 1 year of age because cardiovascular collapse and death can occur [13]. Further precautions should be taken in the use of digoxin because it may act as a proarrhythmic agent in SVT associated with WPW. The long-term management of SVT may include β blockers, procainamide, sotalol, amiodarone, or flecainide. When pharmacologic treatments fail, radiofrequency catheter ablation has an 85% to 95% success rate of preventing recurrence of SVT [21].

The evaluation of SVT includes attempts at elucidating the cause of SVT to prevent future episodes. Laboratory studies may include electrolytes (especially potassium, calcium, magnesium, and glucose), complete blood count, toxicology screen, blood gas, and thyroid function tests. Additionally, creatine kinase and troponins may be added if myocarditis is suspected. Imaging studies can include a chest radiograph (including anteroposterior and lateral views) and an echocardiogram. Once stabilized, the majority of patients who present with SVTs will need to be admitted to a hospital, to investigate the underlying cause of SVT and the potential for long-term medical management or radiofrequency ablation. One could consider safely discharging a patient who has a history of SVT, has presented with minor symptoms such as palpitations, or has had a clear precipitant.

Atrial flutter

Atrial flutter is an uncommon rhythm presenting in the pediatric population. Atrial rates may present in the range of 240 to 450 BPM [4], with the ventricular response depending on the AV nodal conduction. The pacemaker lies in an ectopic focus.

Causes of atrial flutter in children are attributed largely to structural heart disease, including a dilated atria, myocarditis, or acute infection. It is associated most notably with postoperative complications of congenital heart disease repairs, such as atrial septal defect (ASD) repairs, the Mustard procedure for D-transposition of the great arteries, or the Fontan procedure for single ventricle. These procedures cause atrial flutter through disruption in the conduction system, as happens when there is suturing through the atrial septum. Occasionally, patients who have undergone ventricular surgeries such as tetralogy of Fallot repairs may present with atrial arrhythmias. Atrial flutter is also seen in such conditions as Duchenne's muscular dystrophy and central nervous system injury.

On an electrocardiogram, the hallmark pattern is "saw-toothed" flutter waves, which is best viewed in leads II, III, and V1. The atrial rate is, on average, approximately 300 atrial BPM [3]. Because the AV node cannot respond this quickly, there is an AV block, which can present as a 2:1, 3:1, or 4:1 block. The QRS complex is generally normal in configuration (Fig. 5).

Significant cardiac pathology usually accompanies atrial flutter. Because cardiac output is determined by the ventricular rate, with atrial flutter, the ventricular rate is too fast to maintain an efficient cardiac output. Atrial arrhythmias are an important cause of morbidity and mortality in those with congenital heart disease.

Initially, the clinician must recognize whether the patient is hemodynamically stable. An unstable patient may warrant electrical cardioversion, with the con-

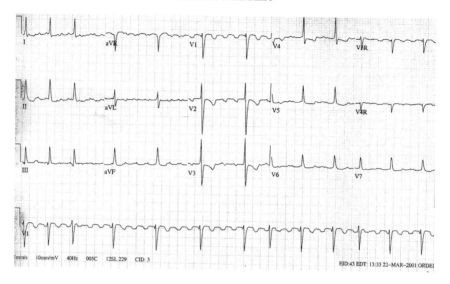

Fig. 5. Atrial flutter. This electrocardiogram is from a child who had undergone a Fontan procedure to repair a hypoplastic left heart. (Courtesy of CDR Jonathan T. Fleenor, MD, Naval Medical Center, San Diego, CA.)

sideration of adding heparin to prevent embolization [3,22]. In patients who are receiving digoxin, it is advisable to avoid electrical cardioversion, unless the condition is life threatening, because the combination is associated with malignant ventricular arrhythmias [23,24]. Alternatives for patients receiving digoxin are rapid atrial pacing with catheterization or lower current settings [22]. For patients who are hemodynamically stable, digoxin is administered to increase AV blockade, thereby slowing the ventricular rate. Propranolol, 1.0 to 4.0 mg/kg/d, orally, divided three to four times daily, may also be added. Recurrences are then prevented, by administering Quinidine.

Atrial fibrillation

Atrial fibrillation is another rare rhythm that presents in children. It is defined as disorganized, rapid atrial activity, with atrial rates ranging from 350 to 600 BPM [11]. The ventricular rate is variable and depends on a varying AV block. The rhythm of atrial fibrillation is described as being "irregularly irregular," alternating between fast and slow rates. On electrocardiography, the hallmark features are irregular atrial waves, with beat-to-beat variability of the atrial size and shape. This is best recognized in lead V1. The QRS complexes appear normal. Children at an increased risk of developing atrial fibrillation include those who have an underlying structural heart defect (such as congenital mitral valve disease and hyperthyroidism) and those who have undergone an intra-atrial operative procedure. Atrial fibrillation is also associated with decreased cardiac output. With a significantly increased ventricular rate, in-coordination ensues between the atria and ventricles, thereby decreasing cardiac output.

When the child presents to the emergency department, the clinician must promptly recognize whether he or she is hemodynamically stable or has cardiac compromise. Hemodynamically unstable patients warrant immediate cardioversion. However, in patients who are hemodynamically stable, digoxin can be administered for ventricular rate control, allowing for a 24-hour time period to assess its efficacy. After that time period elapses and digoxin proves to be ineffective, a second medication may be added such as propranolol, esmolol, or procainamide. In patients who have undergone cardioversion, recurrence is common. During admission, cardioverted patients are often started on an agent to keep them in normal sinus rhythm (eg, amiodarone, procainamide, quinidine, or a β blocker) [25].

Bradydysrhythmias

Bradycardia is defined as a heart rate slower than the lower limit of normal for the patient's age (Table 1), whereas in adults, it is defined as a heart rate less than 60 BPM. Mechanisms of bradycardia include depression of the pacemaker in the sinus node and conduction system blocks. Complete heart block is a common cause of significant bradycardia in pediatric patients and may be acquired or congenital.

Bradycardia in children may be attributable to vagal stimulation, hypoxemia, acidosis, or an acute elevation of intracranial pressure. The most common cause of bradycardia in the pediatric population is hypoxemia. It is important to correct hypoxemia before increasing the heart rate in children.

The management of bradycardia includes the identification of the cause and appropriate cardiopulmonary resuscitation, with assisted ventilation, oxygenation, and chest compressions as indicated. If symptomatic bradycardia persists despite initial resuscitative measures, pharmacologic intervention is initiated with epinephrine (0.01 mg/kg IV; 0.1 mL/kg of 1:10,000 solution) or atropine (0.02 mg/kg, IV, minimum 0.1 mg; maximum single dose is 0.5 mg in children and 1 mg in adolescents). Epinephrine is the initial drug of choice in children with symptomatic bradycardia. Chest compressions are indicated for neonates or children with heart rates less than 60 BPM with hemodynamic compromise [6].

Sinus bradycardia

Sinus bradycardia, includes a heart rate less than the lower limit of normal for the patient's age (see Table 1), with P waves preceding each QRS complex on an EKG. Usually, the heart rate is less than 80 BPM in infants and less than 60 BPM in older children [26]. Sinus bradycardia is a predominantly benign entity, seen most often in athletes and during sleep.

Sinus bradycardia can also be associated with underlying causes. One such ominous cause is an acute onset of increased intracranial pressure as part of Cushing's triad of bradycardia, hypertension, and irregular respirations. An important cause of bradycardia is respiratory compromise. Therefore, the adequacy of the patient's oxygenation and ventilation should be assessed rapidly. Bradycardia can also be associated with hyperkalemia, hypercalcemia, hypoxia, hypothermia, hypothyroidism, and medications (eg, digitalis and β blockers). As with sinus tachycardia, the treatment of sinus bradycardia is targeted at the treatment of the underlying cause.

An important distinction must be made between sinus bradycardia and junctional (nodal) bradycardia. On electrocardiography, junctional bradycardia has either no P waves or inverted P waves after QRS complexes. QRS complexes have a normal configuration and generally have rates between 40 and 60 BPM. Junctional bradycardia may occur in an otherwise normal heart or postoperatively, in cases of digitalis toxicity, or with increased vagal tone. If the patient is asymptomatic, no treatment is indicated. However, if the patient has signs of decreased cardiac output, atropine or pacing may be indicated [4].

Conduction abnormalities

First-degree atrioventricular block

First-degree AV block is an abnormal delay in conduction through the AV node. This type of AV block is a disturbance in the conduction between the normal sinus impulse and its eventual ventricular response. This manifests as a prolonged PR interval on electrocardiography. Meanwhile, the heart is maintained in sinus rhythm, with a normal QRS configuration. There are no dropped beats.

First-degree heart block can be an incidental finding on an otherwise normal EKG reading. Common causes include otherwise healthy children with an infectious disease. It may further be associated with myocarditis (eg, rheumatic fever and Lyme disease), cardiomyopathies, and congenital heart disease (ASD and Ebstein's anomaly).

Second-degree atrioventricular block: Mobitz type I (Wenckebach) and type II

In the Mobitz type I block, otherwise known as the Wenckebach phenomena, the PR interval lengthens progressively until a QRS complex is dropped. This usually occurs over three to six cardiac cycles, followed by a long diastolic pause, and then the cycle resumes. There are occasional and frequent P waves that conduct, and the QRS configuration is normal. The block is caused by an increased refractory period at the level of the AV node. Although this can be seen in otherwise healthy individuals, it can also be seen in patients who have myocarditis, myocardial infarctions, cardiomyopathies, congenital heart disease, digoxin toxicity, and postoperative cardiac repairs.

The Mobitz type II second-degree heart block is known as the "all or none" phenomena. There is either normal AV conduction with a normal PR interval or a completely blocked conduction. The failure of conduction is at the level of the bundle of His, with a prolongation of the refractory period in the His-Purkinje system. Because some of the atrial impulses are not conducted to the ventricle, the ventricular rate depends on the number of conducted atrial impulses.

Third-degree heart block

Third-degree heart block, otherwise known as complete heart block, occurs when none of the atrial impulses is conducted to the ventricles. There is a complete loss of rhythm conduction from a working atrial pacemaker, thereby allowing the ventricular pacemaker to take over. On electrocardiography, the P waves are completely dissociated from the QRS waves. Even though they are dissociated, both the atrial and ventricular rhythms are regular, maintaining regular PP and RR intervals, respectively. The QRS duration is usually normal if the block is usually proximal to the bundle of His, whereas a wide QRS complex indicates that the block is most likely in the bundle branches (eg, surgically induced complete heart block). Oftentimes, the ventricular rhythm is slower than normal (Fig. 6).

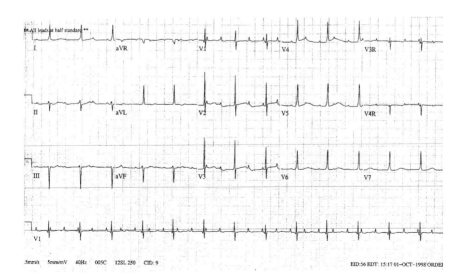

Fig. 6. Complete heart block. This electrocardiogram is from an infant presenting at birth with complete heart block. Note the complete dissociation of P waves from the QRS complexes. The child's mother had systemic lupus erythematosus, which is commonly associated with complete heart block. (Courtesy of CDR Jonathan T. Fleenor, MD, Naval Medical Center, San Diego, CA.)

Complete heart block may be an isolated anomaly. It may also be congenital and is associated with structural lesions, such as in L-transposition of the great arteries and maternal connective tissue disorders. Acquired heart block may result from cardiac surgery, especially when there is suturing in the atrium. This effect can be either transient, resolving within 8 days postoperatively, or permanent. Other causes include infectious causes such as myocarditis, Lyme disease, rheumatic fever, and diphtheria, and inflammatory disorders such as Kawasaki disease and systemic lupus erythematosus. Complete heart block is also associated with myocardial infarction, cardiac tumors, muscular dystrophies, hypocalcemia, and drug overdoses.

Children presenting with first-degree heart block are largely asymptomatic but have the potential to progress to further heart block, including second- and third-degree heart blocks. Those presenting with second-degree, type I (Wenckebach), rarely progress to complete heart block, whereas second-degree, type II, block frequently progresses to complete heart block [4]. Those children who present with complete heart block, most notably in infancy, may present with signs of congestive heart failure. Older children may present with syncopal attacks, otherwise known as Stokes-Adams attacks, with heart rates less than 40 to 45 BPM or even sudden death.

Patients who have complete heart block may present with symptoms related to hypoperfusion, including fatigue, dizziness, impaired exercise tolerance, syncope, confusion, and even sudden death [27]. Acquired or surgically induced heart block generally has a slower ventricular rate, with rates between 40 and 50 BPM, than is seen in congenital heart block, which is generally 50 to 80 BPM [16].

No treatment is indicated for a first-degree degree heart block. However, if suspicious features are present, patients may require evaluation for underlying disease (eg, Lyme disease or rheumatic fever). For second- degree heart blocks, treatment is directed at the underlying cause. In patients who have Mobitz type II second-degree heart block, a prophylactic pacemaker may be warranted because there is a risk of progressing to complete heart block. For those who present with a complete heart block, the mainstay of therapy is a pacemaker. While awaiting pacemaker insertion, it may be necessary to administer atropine or isoproterenol, which temporarily increases the heart rate.

Prolonged QT syndrome

Prolonged QT syndrome, otherwise referred to as long QT syndrome (LQTS), is a disorder of delayed ventricular repolarization, characterized by prolongation of the QT interval, as seen on electrocardiography. Prolongation of the QT interval may be either hereditary or acquired. Jervell-Lange-Nielsen syndrome is an autosomal recessive form of prolonged QT syndrome associated with congenital deafness, whereas Romano-Ward syndrome is an autosomal dominant form that is not associated with deafness. Congenital LQTS, which often presents in childhood, has an estimated incidence of 1 per 10,000 to 1 per 15,000 and is responsible for 3000 to 4000 cases of sudden death each year in the United States. Patients with the acquired type of LQTS usually present in the fifth or sixth decades of life [28]. The most common causes are medications (Box 1) and electrolyte abnormalities such as hypokalemia, hypocalcemia, and hypomagnesemia.

Patients with LQTS commonly present between the ages of 9 and 15 years of age with recurrent episodes of near or frank syncope [29]. Of the patients who have acquired LQTS, 60% of affected individuals are symptomatic at diagnosis [30]. Syncopal episodes are often precipitated by intense emotion, vigorous physical activity, or loud noises. Syncopal episodes may be mistaken for seizures because they can result in the loss of consciousness, tonic-clonic movements, and temporary residual disorientation following the event. A spontaneous return of consciousness usually follows a syncopal episode, but the dysrhythmia has the potential to degenerate into ventricular fibrillation and sudden death. Approximately 10% of children with LQTS present with sudden death, with the youngest children being more likely to die suddenly [31]. LQTS may present in infancy as SIDS or later in life as incidents of near-drowning. Children may also present with milder symptoms such as diaphoresis, palpitations, or lightheadedness.

When a patient presents with syncope, there are a number of historical factors that should be viewed as warning signs of potential cardiac disease and sudden death. Syncope that occurs with exertion is almost always an ominous sign. The strongest risk factors for developing malignant dysrhythmias or sudden death include a history of syncope.

The hallmark dysrhythmia of LQTS, is a polymorphic ventricular tachycardia known as torsades de pointes ("twisting of the points"), a French term first used in 1966 by Dessertenne to describe a QRS axis shifting back and forth around the baseline (Fig. 7) [32]. During this dysrhythmic episode, the cardiac output is markedly impaired, often resulting in syncope or seizures. Although many of these events are self-limiting, with the spontaneous return of consciousness, the dysrhythmia has the potential to degenerate into ventricular fibrillation and

Box 1. Drugs that prolong the qt interval

Antiarrhythmics (class 1A and 3)
Antiemetic (droperidol)
Antifungals (ketoconazole)
Antihistamines (astemizole, terfenidine)
Antimicrobials (erythromycin, trimethoprim-sulfamethoxazole)
Antipsychotics (haloperidol, risperidone)
Organophosphate insecticides
Phenothiazines (thioridazine)
Promotility agents (cisapride)
Tricyclic antidepressants (amitriptyline)

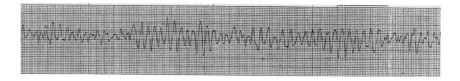

Fig. 7. Rhythm strip of torsades de pointes. This child had a history of dilated cardiomyopathy and returned to sinus rhythm after defibrillation. (Courtesy of CDR Jonathan T. Fleenor, MD, Naval Medical Center, San Diego, CA.)

sudden death. With the potential for fatal consequences in undiagnosed affected individuals, the recognition of LQTS is of paramount importance.

LQTS should be considered and an EKG be obtained on any patient presenting with a suggestive history, including first-degree relatives of known LQTS carrier, a family history of syncope, seizures, sudden death, SIDS, a seizure of unknown cause, or an unexplained near-drowning. Other risk factors include congenital deafness or bradycardia in infants. Suggestive features of syncopal episodes include those that are triggered by emotion, exertion, or stress or those associated with chest pain or palpitations. The QT interval should be measured manually, with lead II generally accepted as being the most accurate. To account for the normal physiologic shortening of the QT interval that occurs with increasing heart rate, the corrected QT interval (QT_c) is calculated using the Bazett formula [33] $QT_c = QT / \sqrt{RR}$. For the greatest accuracy, three consecutive QT intervals and three consecutive preceding RR intervals should be measured and averaged. The current practice identifies a QT_c interval of $\geq$460 ms as prolonged. A QT_c value between 420 and 460 ms is considered borderline and warrants additional assessment [34,35]. Although EKGs automatically calculate the QT and QTc, in patients who have a suggestive history, an EKG with a manual calculation of the QT_c should be performed because the computer calculation often is inaccurate. If the diagnosis of LQTS is suspected but the screening EKG is not diagnostic, increasing sympathetic activity such as with vagal maneuvers may trigger abnormalities on electrocardiography. These abnormalities include QT interval prolongation, prominent U waves, T-wave alternans, and ventricular dysrhythmias (Fig. 8).

Patients presenting with LQTS may require emergency intervention. Patients presenting with an episode of polymorphic ventricular tachycardia or torsades de pointes of unknown origin should receive magnesium (25–50 mg/kg, IV, maximum 2 g). Serum electrolytes and a toxicology screen should be obtained. β blockers may be useful in suppressing catecholamine surges and any further dysrhythmic activity. Patients who exhibit torsades des pointes caused by prolonged QT may worsen acutely, whereas those who have a normal QT interval improve. Patients with recurrent ventricular tachycardia may require temporary transcutaneous ventricular pacing.

Any patient who has a compatible history, a borderline prolongation of the QT interval with symptoms, or an identified prolonged QT syndrome should be referred to a cardiologist for further management. Admission is limited to those

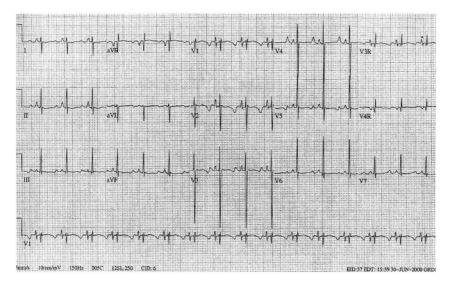

Fig. 8. Long QT interval without associated heart block. A markedly prolonged QT interval is calculated with the Bazett formula [33]: $QTc = QT/\sqrt{}$ preceding RR interval; eg, $QTc = 0.452/\sqrt{0.612}$, then $QTc = 578$ ms. For improved accuracy, average three consecutive RR intervals and three QT intervals, in which each small box $= 0.04$ ms. (Courtesy of CDR Jonathan T. Fleenor, MD, Naval Medical Center, San Diego, CA.)

who are symptomatic or have cardiovascular compromise. Therapy is aimed at reducing sympathetic activity of the heart, either pharmacologically or surgically. β blockers are generally recommended as the initial therapy of choice, which has been shown to effectively eradicate dysrhythmias in 60% of patients and to decrease mortality from 71% in untreated patient to 6% in those who are treated [28,36]. The most commonly used β blockers are propranolol (2–4 mg/kg/d, maximum 60 mg/d) and nadolol (0.5–1 mg/kg/d, maximum 2.5 mg/kg/d). Patients with severe asthma, in whom β blockers are contraindicated, may be candidates for pacemaker therapy.

Once a patient is diagnosed with LQTS, an EKG should be performed on all other family members. All affected individuals regardless of age should be restricted from competitive sports but not necessarily recreational sports. Patients should be educated to avoid triggering factors such as certain medications, loud noises, emotionally stressful situations, and dehydration. Because of the high risk of unexpected cardiac events, family members and close friends should be instructed in CPR and even consider purchasing a home AED.

Summary

In an acute care setting, it is necessary to quickly determine which pediatric ECG findings are normal, which are abnormal, and which must be addressed immediately. A systematic approach to the ECG is essential so that subtle abnormalities are less likely to be missed. A continuous review of the pediatric advanced life support algorithms is imperative in order for the emergency physician to care for children with dysrhythmias.

Acknowledgments

The authors thank CDR Jonathan T. Fleenor, MD, Division of Pediatric Cardiology, Naval Medical Center, San Diego, CA, for electrocardiogram contributions.

References

[1] Sacchetti A, Moyer V, Baricella R, et al. Primary cardiac arrhythmias in children. Pediatr Emerg Care 1999;15:95–8.

[2] Horton L, Mosee S, Brenner J. Use of the electrocardiogram in a pediatric emergency department. Arch Pediatr Adolesc Med 1994;148:184–8.

[3] Park M, Guntheroth W. How to read pediatric ECGs. 3rd edition. St. Louis (MO): Mosby Year Book; 1992.

[4] Park M, George R. Pediatric cardiology for practitioners. 4th edition. St. Louis (MO): Mosby; 2002.

[5] Robinson B, Anisman P, Eshagh E. A primer on pediatric ECGs. Contemp Pediatr 1994;11:69.

[6] Hazinski M, Zaritsky A, Nadkarini V, et al. PALS provider manual. Dallas (TX): American Heart Association; 2002.

[7] Hanna C, Greenes D. How much tachycardia in infants can be attributed to fever? Ann Emerg Med 2004;43:699–705.

[8] Samson R, Berg R, Binghan R. Use of automated external defibrillators for children: an update: an advisory statement from the Pediatric Advanced Life Support Task Force, International Liaison Committee on Resuscitation. Resuscitation 2003;57:237–43.

[9] Cummins RO, Hazinski MF. Guidelines 2000 for cardiopulmonary resuscitation and emergency cardiovascular care: international consensus on science, the major new ECC and CPR guidelines. Circulation 2000;112–28, 291–342.

[10] Dubin D. Rapid interpretation on EKGs. 6th edition. Tampa (FL): COVER Publishing; 2000.

[11] Gewitz MH, Woolf PK. Cardiac emergencies. In: Fleisher G, Ludwig S, editors. Textbook of pediatric emergency medicine. 5th edition. Philadelphia: Lippincott Williams & Wilkins; 2005. p. 717–58.

[12] McEvoy G. Cardiovascular drugs: antiarrhythmic agents. In: AHFS Drug information. Bethesda (MD): American Society of Health-System Pharmacists, Inc.; 2004.

[13] Perry J. Supraventricular tachycardia. In: Garson Jr A, Bricker J, Fisher D, et al, editors. The science and practice of pediatric cardiology. Baltimore (MD): Lippincott Williams & Wilkins; 1998.

[14] Perry J, Garson Jr A. Supraventricular tachycardia due to Wolff Parkinson White syndrome in children: early disappearance and late recurrence. J Am Coll Cardiol 1990;16:1215–20.

[15] Chauhan V, Krahn A, Klein G, et al. Cardiac arrhythmias: supraventricular tachycardia. Med Clin North Am 2001;85:193–223.

[16] Gajewski KK. Cardiology. In: Robertson J, Shilkofski N, editors. Johns Hopkins the Harriet Lane Handbook: a manual for pediatric house officers. 17th edition. St. Louis (MO): Mosby; 2005. p. 159–209.

[17] Losek J, Endom E, Dietrich A, et al. Adenosine and pediatric supraventricular tachycardia in the emergency department: multicenter study and review. Ann Emerg Med 1999;33:185–91.
[18] Vane PD. Cordarone I.V. (amiodarone HCl) prescribing information: precautions, pediatric use of amiodarone. Philadelphia: Wyeth-Ayerst Pharmaceuticals; 2001.
[19] Perry J, Fenrich A, et al. Pediatric use of amiodarone: efficacy and safety in critically ill patients from a multicenter protocol. J Am Coll Cardiol 1996;27:1246–50.
[20] Taketomo CK, Hodding JH, Kraus DM. Pediatric dosage handbook. 9th edition. Hudson (OH): Lexi-Comp, Inc.; 2002–2003. p. 439–40, 916–8.
[21] Danford D, Kugler J, Deal B. The learning curve for radiofrequency ablation of tachyarrhythmias in pediatric patients. Am J Cardiol 1991;18:356–65.
[22] Cummins R, Field J, Hazinski M, et al. ACLS provider manual. Dallas (TX): American Heart Association; 2003.
[23] Ditchey R, Karliner J. Safety of electrical cardioversion in patients without digitalis toxicity. Ann Intern Med 1981;95:676–9.
[24] Ali N, Dais K, Banks T, et al. Titrated electrical cardioversion in patients on digoxin. Clin Cardiol 1982;5:417–9.
[25] Balaji S, Harris L. Atrial arrhythmias in congenital heart disease. Cardiol Clin 2002;20:459–68.
[26] Behrman R, Kliegman R, Jenson H. Cardiac arrhythmias. In: Behrman R, editor. Nelson textbook of pediatrics. 16th edition. Philadelphia: WB Saunders; 2000. p. 1343–61.
[27] Gomes J, Sherif NE. Atrioventricular block: mechanism, clinical presentation, and therapy. Med Clin North Am 1984;68:955–67.
[28] Schwartz P, Periti M, Malliani A. The long QT syndrome. Am Heart J 1975;89:378–90.
[29] Garson A, Dick M, Fournier A, et al. The long QT syndrome in children: an international study of 287 patients. Circulation 1993;87:1866–72.
[30] Ackerman M. The long QT syndrome: ion channel diseases of the heart. Mayo Clin Proc 1998;73:250–69.
[31] Moss A. Prolonged QT interval syndromes. JAMA 1986;256:2985–7.
[32] Dessertenne F. La tachycardia ventriculaire a deux foyers opposes variables [Ventricular tachycardia with 2 variable opposing foci]. Arch Mal Coeur 1966;59:263–72.
[33] Bazett H. An analysis of the time- relations of electrocardiograms. Heart 1920;7:353–70.
[34] Miller M, Porter C, Ackerman M. Diagnostic accuracy of screening electrocardiograms in long QT syndrome. Pediatrics 2001;108:8–12.
[35] Schwartz P, Moss A, Vincent G, et al. Diagnostic criteria for the long QT syndrome, an update. Circulation 1993;88:782–4.
[36] Schwartz P. Idiopathic long QT syndrome: progress and questions. Am Heart J 1985;109:399–411.

ELSEVIER
SAUNDERS

PEDIATRIC CLINICS

OF NORTH AMERICA

Pediatr Clin N Am 53 (2006) 107–137

Abdominal Pain in Children

Maureen McCollough, MD, MPH[a],*, Ghazala Q. Sharieff, MD[b]

[a]*Pediatric Emergency Medicine, Keck USC School of Medicine, 755 Woodward Boulevard, Pasadena, CA 91107, USA*
[b]*Children's Hospital and Health Center, University of California, San Diego, 3030 Children's Way, San Diego, CA 92123, USA*

Abdominal pain and gastrointestinal (GI) symptoms, such as vomiting or diarrhea, are common chief complaints in young children presenting in emergency departments (ED). It is the emergency physician's role to differentiate between a self-limited process such as viral gastroenteritis or constipation and more life-threatening surgical emergencies. Extra-abdominal conditions such as pneumonia or pharyngitis caused by streptococcal infection also can present with abdominal pain and must be considered (Box 1). Considering the difficulties inherent in the pediatric examination, it is not surprising that the diagnoses of appendicitis, intussusception, or malrotation with volvulus continue to be among the most elusive diagnoses for the emergency physician (EP). This article reviews self-limited and more benign gastrointestinal conditions such as viral gastroenteritis or constipation and emergency surgical conditions that may present such as appendicitis or intussusception.

General approach to the child who has abdominal pain

Important information often can be elicited even before speaking to the parents or laying hands on a child. Infants and young toddlers are usually afraid of strangers. Older children may associate a clinic environment or a "man in a white coat" with immunizations and pain. The difficulty of physical examination increases when the physician enters the examination room and the child bursts

* Corresponding author.
E-mail address: mmccollo@usc.edu (M. McCollough).

Box 1. Extra-abdominal causes of gastrointestinal distress

Abdominal epilepsy
Abdominal migraine
Black widow spider bite
Hemolytic uremic syndrome
Henoch-Schöenlein purpura
Ingestions (eg, iron)
Pharyngitis (especially induced by streptococcal infection)
Pneumonia
Sepsis

---

into tears. Observing the child's behavior before any interaction may reveal the reassuring signs of a young child ambulating comfortably around the ED or of an older infant sitting up on a gurney, interested in the surroundings. An older child who walks slowly down a corridor in the ED holding his right lower quadrant similarly has given the examiner a great deal of information. Once the child is approached, use of a nonthreatening manner may pay dividends during the assessment; for example, a position sitting down or kneeling will bring the examiner closer to the child's eye level and is less intimidating.

If a child is found to be poorly responsive or displays other signs of shock, the ongoing assessment of the abdomen will need to occur simultaneously with the immediate priorities of resuscitation. A patent and secure airway must be ensured. Ventilation should be assisted if necessary and supplemental oxygen delivered. Vascular access should be achieved using the intravenous or intraosseous routes, and fluid boluses of normal saline should be administered as necessary. The child should be placed on a cardiac monitor. Immediate bedside tests should include a blood glucose test and hemoglobin determination. The delivery of intravenous antibiotics should not be delayed if there is a reasonable suspicion of underlying sepsis.

Children and parents are often poor historians. Trying to elicit the chronology of symptoms with questions such as "did the pain start before the vomiting or visa versa?" may be difficult. Parents of young infants may only describe their child as irritable and not realize that the abdomen is the source of pain. Adolescents may be embarrassed to talk about bodily functions or sexual issues, especially with physicians of the opposite sex. It is important also to question adolescents about their medical history separately from their parents because they may be more forthcoming when assured of their privacy.

Attempting to bond with the child or using a toy as a distraction before auscultation or palpation can often improve the reliability of the abdominal examination. Infants may be distracted by a set of car keys. Hand and finger puppets also can be used for this purpose. Allowing the child to remain in a parent's arms or lap for as long as possible is also helpful. For older children, examining the mother first may show the child that the examination is nothing to be feared. An older child also can be allowed to place his or her hand on top of the examiner's and simultaneously apply pressure and can be questioned about school or play activities.

Before touching the patient's abdomen, the examiner should look for any obvious abnormalities such as distension, masses, or peristaltic waves. If a child is crying, it should be remembered that the abdomen is relatively soft during the child's' inhalation. This may be the best time to detect masses. To elicit areas of tenderness or peritoneal signs, a quieter, calm child is helpful. If the examiner has difficulty, in some cases it may be possible to have the mother gently push on different areas of the abdomen, while the examiner merely observes the child's response. Another technique is to have the mother hold the child over her shoulder with the child facing away. The examiner can then stand behind the child and slip a hand between the mother and child to palpate the abdomen. Peritoneal signs may also be elicited by having the mother bounce the child up and down on her lap. Fussiness or crying while this maneuver is performed raises the suspicion of peritonitis. Older children can be asked simply to jump up and down.

Rectal examinations are not imperative in a child presenting with abdominal pain. In particular, rectal examinations have not been shown to be helpful in the diagnosis of appendicitis. Rectal examinations, however, can aid in the diagnosis of gastrointestinal bleeding, intussusception, rectal abscess, or impaction. If a rectal examination is necessary, it can be performed by partially introducing a small finger. Inspection of the genitalia may reveal a hair tourniquet, hernia, or signs of testicular torsion and is an important part of the examination.

A thorough extra-abdominal examination is indicated in most children with abdominal pain. For example, failure to examine the throat may lead to a missed diagnosis of pharyngitis, which may be associated with abdominal pain. Lower lobe pneumonias also can mimic an abdominal emergency. The general examination also includes an assessment of the child's hydration status. Classic signs and symptoms of dehydration in infants and young children are dry mucous membranes, decreased tearing, sunken eyes and fontanelles, decreased skin turgor, prolonged capillary refill, and decreased urine output. Interestingly, most of these signs have not been well studied, and some may not be reliable.

For the surgical disease processes discussed in this article, pain is typically the chief complaint. Management of the child's pain during the evaluation is of paramount importance. The use of pain medication in children with abdominal pain does not appear to increase the risk of misdiagnosis [1]. In fact, often a better physical examination can be accomplished once the patient's pain has been addressed.

Gastroenteritis

Epidemiology

Acute gastroenteritis (AGE) is the most common gastrointestinal inflammatory process in children. The cause is usually viral, and rotavirus is the most common virus. In the United States, 200,000 children are hospitalized every year, and 300 to 400 deaths are caused by diarrheal disease. Costs to health care are estimated at $2 billion per year. Rotavirus is the most significant cause of severe diarrhea in childhood, with a peak incidence between 4 and 23 months of age. A rotavirus vaccine was to be part of the routine immunization schedule recommended by the American Academy of Pediatrics; however, the Centers for Disease Control and Prevention does not recommend the vaccine as of 1999 because of the significant number of bowel obstructions and intussusception cases that occurred after the first vaccines were administered. Further studies are underway and may be promising for a new vaccine. Norwalk virus is responsible for up to 40% of diarrheal disease in older children. *Campylobacter* is the leading cause of bacterial diarrhea in the United States.

Presentation

Vomiting usually precedes the diarrhea by as much as 12 to 24 hours. A low-grade fever may or may not be associated with AGE. When the parent states that the child is vomiting "everything," clarify how much the child is taking in at one time (many times a child will drink too much at one time and then vomit). Children who are mildly dehydrated may not manifest clinical signs. Decreased urine output can be a late sign of dehydration. The children who are more at risk for dehydration include those who are younger than 12 months old; those with frequent stools (more than 8 per day); those with frequent vomiting (more than twice per day); and those who are severely undernourished. Examination of the abdomen usually reveals a nondistended soft abdomen with no localized tenderness (may be diffusely, mildly tender), and usually there is minimal to no guarding. AGE may cause an ileus in severe cases.

Viral diarrhea will target the small bowel, resulting in midabdominal cramping and large volumes of watery diarrhea. Bacterial diarrhea will target the large bowel, resulting in lower abdominal pain and smaller volumes of bloody mucoid diarrhea. A bacterial cause should be considered in any child who has a history of travel, has been exposed to an epidemic in daycare, or has higher fevers, bloody stools, or severe cramping. Other diagnoses to consider when a child presents with vomiting include urinary tract infection, appendicitis, inborn errors of metabolism, or volvulus, especially in very young infants, diabetic keto-acidosis, and hemolytic uremic syndrome (the appearance of illness in children usually is preceded by diarrhea).

The assessment of dehydration can be based on the known pre-illness weight in kilograms. The problem in the ED is that parents rarely know the exact weight of a child, especially in kilograms, and scales may vary slightly. If the pre-illness weight is known, then every kilogram of weight lost corresponds to a loss of 1 L of body fluid. The assessment of dehydration also can be based on clinical findings. The percentage of dehydration based on clinical findings such as dry mucous membranes or decreased urine output can vary slightly from reference

Table 1
Clinical signs and percentages of dehydration

Age and sign	Dehydration		
	Mild	Moderate	Severe
Older child	3% (30 cc/kg)	6% (60 cc/kg)	9% (90 cc/kg)
Infant	5% (50 cc/kg)	5–10% (100 cc/kg)	≥ 10%
Clinical sign			
Touch of skin	Normal	Dry	Clammy
Skin turgor	Normal	Tenting	None
Mucosa	Moist	Dry	Parched
Eyes	Normal	Deep set	Sunken
Tears	Present	Decreased	None
Fontanelle	Flat	Soft	Sunken
Central nervous system	Consolable	Irritable	Lethargic/obtunded
Heart rate	Regular	Increased	Very increased
Urine output	Normal	Decreased	None

to reference. When clinical signs of dehydration are found in infants, the infants will have a higher percentage of dehydration than in older children (Table 1). The more clinical signs of dehydration the child has, the higher the percentage of dehydration will be [2,3].

Laboratory and radiology findings

A blood glucose check is recommended if the vomiting or abdominal pain is prolonged or associated with polyuria or polydipsia, to rule out diabetic ketoacidosis. Hypoglycemia in an alert child is generally not a concern [4]. Electrolytes generally do not need to be checked in well-appearing children who have signs of mild dehydration. The American Academy of Pediatrics (AAP) does not recommend electrolytes in every child; rather, the AAP recommends electrolytes in children who have acute gastroenteritis with, among other signs, an altered mental status, clinical signs of moderate to severe dehydration, clinical signs of hypernatremia or hypokalemia, prolonged, severe diarrhea (≥ 48 hours) as a risk for hypokalemia, infants who are ≤ 6 months old, and suspicious or unusual histories. The bicarbonate level has not been shown to be well correlated with the degree of dehydration.

A urinalysis to rule out infection is recommended, especially in young females who present only with abdominal pain and vomiting. A young infant who has vomiting and clinical signs of dehydration without ketones in the urine may have an inborn error of metabolism. Stool cultures generally are not necessary in most children who present with vomiting and diarrhea. Cultures should be considered in cases of admission, systemic illness, travel history, daycare exposure, a food- or water-borne source, recent antibiotics, bloody or mucoid stools, immunocompromised infants, or epidemics.

Management

Children with clinical signs of dehydration need rehydration. Rehydration can be administered either orally or through a nasogastric tube or an intravenous line. If a child has signs of severe dehydration, altered mental status, or evidence of an ileus, then rehydration should occur through an intravenous line.

An oral challenge is not oral rehydration. If a child is going to be orally rehydrated, then parents need to be instructed on the proper techniques of oral rehydration. Oral rehydration is very effective but is more labor intensive for children and parents [5]. However, when surveyed, parents actually prefer oral rehydration compared with intravenous rehydration. The commercially available rehydration solutions (eg, Pedialyte or Rehydralyte) are fairly close to delivering the optimal amount of sodium and glucose recommended by the World Health Organization (sodium plus 60–90 mEq and dextrose 2.0%). Many homemade recipes (eg, a water, salt, and sugar mixture) for oral rehydration solution can be found on the Internet.

The key to successful oral rehydration in children who present with vomiting is to offer small amounts at a time; for example, 5 cc (sips) for young children or 15 cc (tablespoon) for older children every 2 minutes. A syringe or a 5-F feeding tube attached to a syringe can be used to help facilitate the oral rehydration. The parent also can drip the solution slowly into the child's mouth or through the nares into the posterior pharynx. If vomiting occurs, wait 10 to 15 minutes and try again. The child should receive either 50 cc/kg orally for mild to moderate dehydration or 100 cc/kg for moderate to severe dehydration, over 3 to 4 hours. Children who experience ongoing losses, such as by continued diarrhea, should receive an additional 10 cc/kg of rehydration.

Breast feeding infants can be rehydrated using more frequent, shorter feeds. Another option for oral rehydration is the use of frozen rehydration popsicles such as Revital-ICE. Placing a nasogastric tube is an alternative route for hydration in the child who refuses absolutely to take anything by mouth or in whom an intravenous line cannot be established but is clinically stable [6].

Intravenous rehydration should be used for any child who fails oral rehydration or has signs of severe dehydration, an ileus, or an altered mental status. Many experts recommend a minimum of 30 to 40 cc/kg in cases of mild to moderate dehydration, which will correct dehydration of 3% to 4%. Antiemetics and antidiarrheal medications are not recommended currently by the AAP because of limited literature to support their use [7]. Prochlorperazine, promethazine, and metoclopramide have been shown to be of some benefit but have some increased risk of sedation and an increased risk of dystonic reaction in children. However, many emergency and pediatric emergency physicians understand that is cruel to allow a child to remain nauseous and vomiting in the ED. Ondansetron (Zofran), a 5-hydroxytryptamine-3 receptor antagonist, which has been used for years as chemotherapy for pediatric nausea, has now been studied in emergency departments for children with acute gastroenteritis [8,9]. More literature is needed to support the use of antidiarrheal agents in children, but many emergency physicians use these medications in otherwise healthy older children who are presumed to have viral diarrhea.

Live bacterial cultures, such as *Lactobacillus* in yogurt, have been shown to help treat infectious diarrhea and to help prevent diarrhea associated with antibiotics [10]. Antibiotics are not recommended for most children who are presumed to have viral AGE. In children with confirmed bacterial diarrhea, the role of antibiotics in treating infections by *Campylobacter jejuni*, *Escherichia coli*, and *Yersinia* is unclear. Nontyphoid *Salmonella* infection is self-limiting and may have prolonged excretion with antibiotic therapy. However, the treatment for *Salmonella* is indicated in infants less than 3 months of age, who have a history of immunodeficiency or hemoglobinopathy. Antibiotic therapy should not be initiated unless *E coli* 0157:H7 has been excluded because patients may develop hemolytic uremic syndrome from empiric antibiotic use. *Shigella* infection may be treated with trimethoprim-sulfamethoxazole, 8 mg/kg/d, divided twice per day, or erythromycin, 40 mg/kg/d, divided four times per day, for 5 to 7 days. Erythromycin is the drug of choice for treating *Campylobacter* infection. *Giardia* may be treated with metronidazole, 15 mg/kg/d, divided three times per day, for 7 days. *Clostridium difficile* infections may be treated with oral vancomycin, 50 mg/kg/d, divided four times per day, or metronidazole for 7 days.

Resuming formula feeding in young infants or solids in older children as soon as possible should also be encouraged. Transient lactose intolerance may develop, especially during AGE caused by rotavirus, but is transient. Most children can return to eating milk products or formula. Occasionally, lactose intolerance persists and may be a cause of post-AGE diarrhea. If persistent diarrhea occurs after the reintroduction of milk products or if the stool is acidic and contains more than 0.5% reducing substances, a lactose-free formula should be considered.

Constipation

Parents often worry that their infant or child is constipated, particularly because it is common for infants to strain and turn red in the face during bowel movements. Unfortunately, a uniform definition of constipation has yet to be determined. The best way is to define constipation is not by the frequency of the stool but by the difficulty or painful passage of large or hard stools. Newborns typically have a meconium stool in the first 48 hours of life and then can range from zero to 12 stools per day for the first week of life. The stools of breast-fed infants are very soft and pale yellow and often occur after each feeding. However, bottle-fed infants tend to have firm, formed, yellow stools one to four times per day. When infants are 3 to 4 months of age, stool frequency decreases, with some bottle-fed infants passing one stool every other day. Most children develop the adult pattern of having a mean of 1.2 stools per day by 4 years of age.

Causes

The more common serious causes of constipation in the newborn and infant are imperforate anus, anal stenosis, meconium plug syndrome, meconium ileus, Hirschsprung's disease, volvulus, anal fissure, infant botulism, hypocalcemia, hypercalcemia, and hypothyroidism. Constipation in the older infant or child is related commonly to changes in diet, especially from breast milk to formula or advancement to solid baby foods. Inadequate fluid intake is another common cause of constipation. The school-aged child may present with constipation caused by high carbohydrate diets and a hesitance to go to the bathroom at school. The child who has rectal retention and encopresis has fecal soiling of the underpants and may paradoxically complain of diarrhea. A lower abdominal mass may be found by palpation, and fecal impaction may be found on rectal examination. Older children may present with abdominal pain, which may be in the right lower quadrant and mimic appendicitis.

Presentation

Pertinent history that should be obtained from the caregiver includes the time after birth of the first bowel movement, frequency of bowel movements, consistency and size of stools, presence of pain with bowel movements, and associated systemic findings such as fever, weight loss, and vomiting. Dietary habits should be a particular focus, and a medication history should also be obtained. A complete physical examination should be performed, including an abdominal palpation for masses, inspection of the perineum and perianal area for fissures, and imperforate anus or stenosis. A plain abdominal radiograph is helpful in confirming the diagnosis when the history or physical examination is confusing or inconclusive.

Laboratory and radiologic findings

Laboratory tests and radiologic studies generally are unnecessary in the diagnosis and management of constipation in young children. An abdominal series or flat-plate radiograph of the abdomen can confirm that the colon has a significant amount of stool present.

Management

If fecal impaction is present, disimpaction is necessary. Oral medications include mineral oil, 1 to 4 mL/kg/dose, once or twice per day (contraindicated in infants and in children at risk for aspiration); lactulose, 1 to 2 mL/kg/dose, once or twice per day; milk of magnesia, 1 to 3 mL/kg/dose, once or twice per day, or with medications containing polyethylene glycol (PEG); or sorbitol, senna, or bisacodyl [11]. A tasteless, commercially available electrolyte-free PEG solution (MiraLax) can be mixed with any clear liquid beverage [12]. It is prepared by dissolving 1 capful (17 g) of powder in 8 oz of liquid and giving the child 10 to 14 mL/kg/d in two divided doses. Rectal disimpaction also can be performed. However, hypertonic phosphate enemas have been associated with severe, acute hypocalcemia and cardiac arrest in infants [13]. Tap water enemas have been associated with acute hyponatremia, seizures, and death [14]. In the older infant and toddler, milk of magnesia, mineral oil, or lactulose can be used. Docusate (Colace), 5 to 10 mg/kg/d or senna extract (Senokot), 5 to 10 mL daily, can be safely used in older children.

Maintenance therapy of constipation is most appropriately managed by a primary care clinician. Dietary management includes increasing fluid intake and adding fiber and fruits such as prunes, pears, or plums to the diet. A barley extract (Maltsupex) or Karo syrup can be recommended safely for infants in a dosage of 1 to 2 teaspoons two to four times daily, added to formula, juice, or food. Behavioral modification for the older child includes regular toilet sitting, stool diaries, and reward systems. If an anal fissure is discovered, management includes frequent, gentle, thorough cleansing of the anus and liberal lubrication with petroleum jelly. A stool softener must be used, and a topical anesthetic ointment may be helpful to avoid a pattern of pain and stool retention.

Appendicitis

Causes

Appendicitis is the abdominal pain most commonly treated surgically in childhood, affecting four of every 1000 children. Appendicitis is the cause of pain in 2.3% of all the children with abdominal pain seen in ambulatory clinics or EDs. Of all the children admitted to the hospital with abdominal pain, 82% are diagnosed with appendicitis [15]. Because of the difficulty in evaluating young children with abdominal pain, perforation rates for appendicitis are higher than in the general adult population (30%–65%). Moreover, because the omentum is less developed in children, perforations are less likely to be "walled off" or localized, leading to generalized peritonitis.

Presentation

The classic presentation, consisting of generalized abdominal pain migrating to the right lower quadrant, associated with nausea, vomiting, and fever, is seen less often in the pediatric patient [16]. In addition, children often present earlier in their clinical course than adults do, when only mild or less specific symptoms are present. However, limited data appear to indicate that individual signs such as rebound tenderness and Rovsing's sign have a high sensitivity and specificity in children [4].

The most common findings of appendicitis in children are right lower quadrant pain, abdominal tenderness, guarding, and vomiting [17]. If available, a history of abdominal pain preceded by vomiting can be helpful in distinguishing appendicitis from acute gastroenteritis. Very young children commonly have diarrhea as the presenting symptom [18]. Bearing in mind the special techniques discussed above for eliciting peritoneal irritation, the EP should also remember that the position of the appendix can vary greatly, and tenderness may be found in locations other than the classic McBurney point. Although the rectal examination is not usually helpful in making a diagnosis of appendicitis [19], some authors advocate a rectal examination in infants, in whom there may be a palpable rectal mass in up to 30% of cases [20]. Changes in skin temperature over the area of the appendix have not been shown to be helpful in the diagnosis of appendicitis [21].

Differential diagnosis

Gastroenteritis is the most common diagnosis in cases of missed appendicitis. Although enteritis caused by *Y enterocolitica* and *Y pseudotuberculosis* has been termed the "great imitator" of appendicitis, in reality, the amount of diarrhea in gastroenteritis is usually more pronounced. Appendicitis is also frequently mistaken for a urinary tract infection (UTI), which may also present with abdominal pain and vomiting. A study reported by Reynolds [22] in 1993 showed that missed cases of appendicitis were more likely to have diarrhea, to not be anorexic, and to be afebrile.

Laboratory evaluation

No laboratory test is 100% sensitive and specific for appendicitis. The white blood cell count (WBC) can be helpful in the diagnosis, although, by itself, it is neither specific nor sensitive for appendicitis and therefore cannot be used alone to rule in or rule out the disease [23]. The WBC, however, can be used as an adjunct, after the clinical suspicion of appendicitis is estimated. If clinical suspicion is low before any laboratory or other investigations (for example, in a child who has vomiting and diarrhea but minimal abdominal tenderness) and the WBC is normal, the likelihood of appendicitis becomes very low. If the WBC is high, the likelihood of appendicitis is raised sufficiently to warrant further tests or observation.

A urinalysis should be performed; however, caution must be exercised in its interpretation, because mild pyuria, hematuria, and bacteriuria can all be present if an inflamed appendix is located adjacent to a ureter. The presence of C-reactive protein also has been studied as a marker for appendicitis [24–27], but it is not significantly more sensitive or specific than the WBC.

Diagnostic radiology

Plain film abdominal series typically have nonspecific findings and are of low yield in cases of appendicitis [15]. Appendicoliths are present only in approximately 10% of true appendicitis cases. Barium enemas have also been used, with the principle that an inflamed appendix will fail to fill and will not be visualized. Unfortunately, 10% to 30% of normal appendices are not visualized with barium studies, creating a high number of false-positive results [28].

Ultrasonography is considered by many experts to be the imaging test of choice in children. Ultrasonography is noninvasive, rapid, and can be performed at the bedside. It does not require oral contrast, which is an advantage for patients who may require surgery. It also spares the pediatric patient exposure to radiation. The normal appendix in pediatric patients is visualized readily by ultrasonography because there is usually less abdominal wall fat than in adults. Graded compression of the appendix is used to determine the presence or absence of inflammation. An inflamed appendix is usually aperistaltic, difficult to compress, and measures ≥ 6 mm in diameter. It is important for the ultrasonographer to visualize the entire appendix to avoid a false-negative reading because sometimes only the distal tip of the appendix is inflamed. The mucosal lining may be intact or poorly defined, and a fecolith may or may not be present. A periappendiceal fluid collection may indicate an early perforation but may result simply from inflammation. Experienced ultrasonographers can achieve sensitivities of 85% to 90% and specificities of 95% to 100% in acute appendicitis [29–37]. However, studies have not shown an improvement in outcome measures such as a decrease in negative laparotomies or time to the operating room [38,39]. Color flow Doppler ultrasonography is now being added to increase the accuracy of the sonographic examinations. Doppler measurement demonstrates an increase in blood flow to the area of an inflamed appendix [40].

In recent years, CT has become the test of choice for pediatric surgeons when ultrasonography fails to give a definitive diagnosis [41]. Every variation, from triple-contrast (intravenous, oral, and rectal) CT scanning to noncontrast, unenhanced CT, has been used [42,43]. CT offers the advantage of greater accuracy, the ability to identify alternative diagnoses, and in some studies, lower negative laparotomy rates [44]. Although CT appears to be better than ultrasonography in making the diagnosis of appendicitis in children [45], it is slower, requires oral contrast in most centers, and exposes the young child to significant radiation. If the child is vomiting, keeping the oral contrast in the gastrointestinal tract can be a challenge, and antiemetics may be required.

Leukocyte imaging studies [46] and technetium scans [47] have been used for equivocal cases of abdominal pain in children. The overall sensitivity, specificity, and accuracy, however, are lower than with CT. Magnetic resonance imaging is also superior in its ability to diagnose appendicitis in children [48], but it may not be available or practical. No study can be relied on for 100% accuracy. If clinical suspicion is high and imaging studies are negative, the child should be hospitalized for observation and serial examinations.

Management

When the clinical suspicion for appendicitis is high, consultation with a surgeon is warranted before any radiologic study. Nonetheless, many surgeons will request a diagnostic study to decrease the likelihood of a negative laparotomy. When the diagnosis of appendicitis is made, then preparing the child for the operating room is essential. Usually the oral intake of these children has been limited during the day or days before presentation, and intravenous fluids are necessary. Electrolyte imbalances should also be addressed, although significant abnormalities are not common in children with appendicitis.

If there are clinical or radiologic signs of perforation, antibiotics with gram-negative and anaerobic coverage should be started in the ED [49]. A few studies have shown a benefit to antibiotic therapy in decreasing infectious complications in children with uncomplicated, nonperforated appendicitis as well [50]. Diagnosing appendicitis early is the key to a better outcome. Any child who is evaluated in the ED with a chief complaint of abdominal pain and who is considered well enough to go home but in whom the diagnosis of appendicitis has not been ruled out should be asked to return to the ED within 8 hours for another evaluation of the abdomen.

Intussusception

Pathophysiology

Intussusception was first described over 300 years ago. It is the prolapse of one part of the intestine into the lumen of an immediately distal adjoining part. The most common type is ileocolic invagination. During the invagination, the mesentery is dragged along into the distal lumen, and venous return is obstructed. This leads to edema, bleeding of the mucosa, increased pressure in the area, and eventually obstruction to arterial flow. Gangrene and perforation result.

Causes

Intussusception is seen most frequently between the ages of 3 months and 5 years, with 60% of cases occurring in the first year and a peak incidence at 6 to 11 months of age. The disorder, which appears predominantly in males, was once believed to occur more often in the spring and autumn, although now it appears it has no seasonality [51,52]. Although it is usually idiopathic in the younger age groups, children older than 5 years often have a pathologic "lead point" for intussusception, such as polyps, lymphoma, Meckel's diverticulum, or Henoch-Schöenlein purpura and require a work-up to determine the underlying cause.

Presentation

The classic triad of intermittent colicky abdominal pain, vomiting, and bloody mucous stools is encountered in only 20% to 40% of cases. At least two of these findings will be present in approximately 60% of patients. The vomiting is not necessarily bilious because the level of obstruction is low in the ileocecal area. A palpable abdominal mass in the right upper or lower quadrant is an uncommon finding [53].

Abdominal pain associated with intussusception is colicky, lasts for approximately 1 to 5 minutes at a time, and then abates for 5 to 20 minutes. During episodes of pain, the child cries and may draw the knees upward toward the chest. Although the child often looks better between episodes, he or she still usually appears ill, quiet, or exhausted. Gradually, irritability increases and vomiting becomes more frequent and sometimes bilious. Fever may also develop at this point as the child deteriorates.

If a colicky episode is not witnessed by the ED staff, the EP should ask the parents to describe or demonstrate what the child was doing during the episodes. Most parents of a child who has gastroenteritis do not indicate that their child is in pain. Parents of a child who presents with intussusception usually believe that the child is in pain before or during episodes of vomiting. Intussusception also can present with lethargy, pallor, and unresponsiveness. It is important to keep this diagnosis in mind when dealing with an infant who has an altered mental status [54].

The abdomen may be distended and tender, but usually the pain appears to be out of proportion to the physical examination. There may be an elongated mass in the right upper or lower quadrants. Any type of blood in the stool may be caused by intussusception. Rectal examination may reveal either occult blood or frankly bloody, foul-smelling stool, classically described as "currant jelly" [55]. However, frank rectal bleeding is a late and unreliable sign; its absence should not deter the EP in the pursuit of the diagnosis. It should also be noted that what appears to be blood in a child's stool may be something else, such as red fruit punch or Jell-O, therefore, guaiac testing may prevent this error when there is some question. A period of observation in the ED for the recurrence of a pain episode is helpful in equivocal cases. Specifically noting the absence of such episodes during ED observation is good practice and should be documented in the clinical record.

Differential diagnosis

Gastroenteritis presents typically with more diarrhea than intussusception, and the child usually has ill contacts. The presence of any degree of blood in the stool should also raise suspicion for a more serious condition. Bleeding from a Meckel's diverticulum usually is painless, unless the diverticulum becomes inflamed.

An incarcerated hernia or testicular or ovarian torsion may also present with sudden abdominal pain and vomiting. Inspection of the genitalia, especially in males, is vital. With torsion, the rectal examination does not show occult or frank blood. Renal colic presenting with pain and vomiting generally is not seen in young children.

Laboratory tests

No laboratory test reliably rules in or out the diagnosis of intussusception. If the bowel has become ischemic or necrotic, acidosis may be present.

Diagnostic imaging

Unfortunately, plain abdominal films are neither sensitive nor specific for intussusception [56,57]. Plain films initially may appear normal. As the disease progresses, a variety of abnormalities may be seen, including a visible abdominal mass, abnormal distribution of gas and fecal contents, air fluid levels, and dilated loops of small intestine. A "target sign" on plain film consists of concentric circles of fat density, similar in appearance to a doughnut, visualized to the right of the spine. This sign is caused by layers of peritoneal fat surrounding and within the intussusception alternating with layers of mucosa and muscle. Less commonly, the soft tissue mass of the intussusception (leading edge) can be seen projecting into the colon. Large areas of gas with the head of the intussuscepted bowel may take the shape of a crescent, although other patterns may be seen.

Ultrasonography is used in some institutions to diagnose intussusception and to confirm reduction after treatment [58]. Sonographic findings in intussusception include the target sign, a single hypoechoic ring with a hyperechoic center and the "pseudokidney" sign, superimposed hypo- and hyperechoic areas representing the edematous walls of the intussusceptum and layers of compressed mucosa. Doppler flow may be used to identify bowel ischemia. If signs of intussusception are not identified by ultrasonography in cases in which the diagnosis is suspected clinically, proceeding with a barium or air enema should still be considered.

Management

The main focus in the management of a child who has intussusception is emergent reduction of the obstructed bowel. Classically, this reduction is accomplished by a barium enema, which acts as both a diagnostic and therapeutic radiologic study. The barium enema has been the gold standard for both the diagnosis and treatment of intussusception for decades [59]. Saline enemas have also been used successfully [60,61], and newer modalities such as air enemas and ultrasonographically guided enemas have emerged.

Many centers in the United States are now moving toward air enemas [62–67]. This modality was first introduced to the Western world at the American Pediatric Surgical Association meeting in 1985, with the presentation of a series of 6396 successfully treated patients [68]. Air enemas offer several advantages over barium enemas. They are easier to administer, and in most studies, they have a higher rate of successful reduction. Air enemas using fluoroscopic guidance deliver much less radiation than barium studies, and if ultrasonography guidance is used, there is no exposure. Limiting radiation exposure is important to consider when dealing with infants and their susceptible reproductive organs; and if a perforation occurs during these investigations, air is much less dangerous to the peritoneum and abdominal contents than barium is.

Visualization of the entire colon to the terminal ileum is mandatory to rule out ileocolic intussusception. Ileo–ileo intussusception can be much harder to diagnose and much harder to reduce. Spontaneous reduction of intussuscepted bowel has been reported, although in a patient with significant symptoms, therapeutic intervention should not be delayed [69].

Not every child who has intussusception should undergo bowel reduction by enema. Clinical signs of peritonitis, perforation, or hypovolemic shock are clear contraindications to enemas. These signs mandate surgical exploration. Relative contraindications to enemas include prolonged symptoms (≥ 24 hours), evidence of obstruction such as air fluid levels on plain abdominal films, and ultrasonography findings of intestinal ischemia or trapped fluid.

Even in well-selected patients, enemas may cause the reduction of necrotic bowel, perforation, and sepsis. After a successful reduction, the child should be admitted for observation. A small percentage of patients (0.5%–15%) will have a recurrence of the intussusception, usually within 24 hours but sometimes after days or weeks. Even after reduction by laparotomy, the recurrence rate is 2% to 5% [52].

Small bowel obstruction

Pathophysiology

Small bowel obstruction may result from intrinsic, extrinsic, or intraluminal disease. Although the most common causes of small bowel obstruction are adhesions from previous abdominal surgery and incarceration of a hernia [70], intussusception, appendicitis, Meckel's diverticulum, malrotation with midgut volvulus, and tumors also should be considered as possible causes. In addition to inguinal hernias, umbilical, obturator, and femoral canal hernias may also lead to small bowel obstruction [56].

Presentation

As obstruction develops, decreased oral intake occurs and vomiting ensues, often becoming bilious in nature. This is followed by obstipation. Abdominal distension and tenderness occur, and the abdomen may be tympanic to percussion. If the small bowel obstruction is caused by mechanical compression, high-pitched bowel sounds with "rushes" may be heard. When intraluminal pressure becomes higher than the venous and arterial pressures, ischemia develops in the bowel, and hematochezia may be seen. As with most abdominal emergencies in children, hematochezia is a late finding. Sepsis is another late finding because bacteria from the ischemic bowel enter the blood.

Differential diagnosis

Abdominal pain and vomiting also can be seen with other processes such as appendicitis. As time passes, a bowel obstruction will develop more abdominal distension than is seen typically in other processes. The lack of stool or gas passage points toward bowel obstruction. It is important to remember that the underlying cause of the obstruction may be as important to recognize as the obstruction itself.

Laboratory tests

No laboratory test is diagnostic of a bowel obstruction. Elevated levels of blood urea nitrogen, creatinine, and hematocrit may signify dehydration.

Diagnostic radiology

Plain abdominal films should be obtained when obstruction is suspected. A paucity of air in the abdomen is the most common finding in young children with bowel obstruction. Distended loops of bowel may be seen; however, smooth bowel walls are more common than distended bowel in small children. Multiple air–fluid levels also are seen commonly with small bowel obstruction. In later presentations, the bowel may resemble a tangle of hoses or sausages. An upright or lateral decubitus film will help to determine whether free air is present, caused by perforation. Further study with ultrasonography, CT, an upper-GI series, or an enema should be performed when there is suspicion of underlying pathologies such as appendicitis, midgut volvulus, and intussusception.

Management

Immediate surgical consultation is indicated when a bowel obstruction is seen on plain radiographs. Morbidity and mortality are increased if the obstruction is not treated within 24 hours [71]. The patient should be aggressively hydrated with normal saline boluses, and a nasogastric tube should be placed for gastric decompression. Broad-spectrum antibiotics are indicated, particularly if peritonitis is suspected.

Incarcerated hernia

Causes

Inguinal hernias occur in 1% to 4% of the population, more often in males (6:1), and more often on the right side (2:1). Premature infants are at a higher risk for hernias (30%), and 60% of incarcerated inguinal hernias occur during the first year of life. Umbilical hernias are also commonly seen in the infant population. Unlike inguinal hernias, umbilical hernias will rarely become incarcerated and usually will close without surgery by 1 year of age. Other disorders place patients at an increased risk for abdominal hernias, including ventriculoperitoneal shunts, peritoneal dialysis, Marfan's syndrome, cystic fibrosis, mucopolysaccharidoses, and hypospadias.

Presentation

Hernias usually present with an asymptomatic bulge in the groin or umbilical area, made more prominent with crying, straining, or laughing. The first sign of incarceration of an inguinal hernia is an abrupt onset of irritability in the young infant. Refusal to eat soon follows, followed by vomiting, which may become bilious and sometimes feculent.

Inguinal hernias may be palpated as smooth, firm, sausage-shaped, mildly tender masses in the groin; the hernia originates proximal to the inguinal ring and can extend into the scrotum. The "silk glove sign" occurs when the index finger rubs over the proximal spermatic cord and sometimes two layers of hernial sac can be felt rubbing together. If the child appears to be well, without vomiting, fever, or redness to the inguinal area, then the hernia is not likely incarcerated.

Differential diagnosis

There are many conditions that may mimic an inguinal hernia, but the most common condition is a hydrocele. A hydrocele is the result of incomplete obliteration of the process vaginalis, which allows an out-pocketing of peritoneum to appear in the scrotum. This fluid-filled sac can appear anywhere from the spermatic cord to the testicle, and if it is large, it can be transilluminated. Hydroceles can be palpated separately from the testes and are freely movable. A hydrocele usually appears in the first few months of life and disappears by 1 year of age.

Diagnostic imaging

If the diagnosis is uncertain, a scrotal ultrasonogram can differentiate an inguinal hernia from a hydrocele.

Management

If signs of incarceration are not present, a reduction should be attempted in the ED. Reduction of the hernia can be accomplished usually by placing the child in Trendelenburg position with ice packs to the area and the administration of pain medication. If reduction is not possible or if the hernia appears incarcerated or ischemic, emergent surgical consultation is required. Umbilical hernias rarely will become incarcerated and often will close without surgery.

Meckel's diverticulum

Pathophysiology and causes

Meckel's diverticulum is the most common congenital abnormality of the small intestine. Meckel's diverticulum is a remnant of the omphalomesenteric (vitelline) duct that disappears normally by the seventh week of gestation. It is a true diverticulum, containing all layers of the bowel wall. Up to 60% of these diverticuli containing heterotopic gastric tissue and heterotopic pancreatic, endometrial, and duodenal mucosa have also been reported [72,73]. The features of Meckel's diverticulum are commonly described by "the rule of 2s" [70]: it is present in approximately 2% of the population with only 2% of affected patients becoming symptomatic. Forty-five percent of symptomatic patients are less than 2 years of age [74]. The most common location is 2 feet (40–100 cm) from the ileocecal valve, and the diverticulum typically is 2 inches long.

Clinical presentation

The classic presentation of Meckel's diverticulum is painless or minimally painful rectal bleeding. Isolated, red rectal bleeding is common, particularly in boys less than 5 years of age [75]. Such painless bleeding is a result of heterotopic gastric tissue in the diverticulum or in the adjacent ileum. Abdominal pain, distension, and vomiting may occur if obstruction has occurred, and the presentation may mimic appendicitis or diverticulitis. Meckel's diverticulum may also ulcerate and perforate, presenting as a bowel perforation, or act as a lead point, resulting in intussusception.

Differential diagnosis

The differential diagnosis includes both painful and nonpainful conditions. Rectal bleeding associated with abdominal pain may be caused by peptic ulcer disease, intussusception, and volvulus. Nonpainful rectal bleeding may be caused by polyps, arteriovenous malformations, and tumors.

Laboratory tests

Although no laboratory test is diagnostic of Meckel's diverticulum, children with gastrointestinal bleeding should undergo screening laboratory tests such as a complete blood count, coagulation profile, and a type and screen.

Diagnostic radiology

Abdominal films may show signs of obstruction such as dilated loops of bowel or a paucity of bowel gas. Scanning Meckel's diverticulum involves an intravenous injection of technetium-pertechnetate. This test relies on the presence of gastric mucosa in or near the diverticulum that has an affinity for the radionucleotide. A scan of Meckel's diverticulum can detect the presence of gastric mucosa within the diverticulum with up to 85% accuracy [76]. Mesenteric arteriography can detect the site of active bleeding if bleeding is profuse.

Management

As carried out in any patient with active bleeding, fluid resuscitation is warranted, starting with boluses of normal saline, 20 cc/kg. A blood transfusion may be necessary, with a packed red blood cell increment of 10 cc/kg. The patient should have nothing by mouth, and a nasogastric tube should be placed. Antibiotic therapy must be initiated if there are peritoneal signs. Surgical consultation should be obtained emergently. Surgical intervention may involve a diverticulectomy or a more extensive small bowel segmental resection if there is irreversible bowel ischemia.

Very young infants

Very young infants, those less than a few months old, also have unique gastrointestinal conditions. Colic should be considered a diagnosis of exclusion. Hypertrophic pyloric stenosis is a common presentation, and surgical correction does not need to be immediate. Volvulus caused by congenital malrotation is a true surgical emergency, and consultation with a pediatric surgeon should be immediate once the diagnosis is considered. Fortunately, necrotizing entero-colitis, another gastrointestinal condition of newborns with serious sequelae, is usually seen by pediatric colleagues in the newborn nursery or neonatal intensive care unit.

Colic

Colic affects 1 in 6 families and is more likely to be reported by older mothers with longer full-time education and nonmanual occupations. To this day, the cause of colic remains unclear but is believed to be related to increased gas production in the infant's intestines and, possibly, to neurologic or psychologic reasons. Other experts consider colic to be part of the normal distribution of crying.

Presentation

Colic appears usually during the second week of life and is characterized by screaming episodes and a distended or tight abdomen; some infants will draw up their legs, pass gas, cry, and act miserable for hours. Episodes may last minutes to hours, occurring usually in the evening. One common definition used is 3 hours per day, 3 days per week, and at least 3 weeks in duration. Severity can increase around 4 to 8 weeks of age and will usually resolve around 12 weeks of age.

Growth and development remain unchanged, and the physical examination is unremarkable. No vomiting, diarrhea, fever, or weight loss occurs with colic. For any inconsolable crying infant, other correctable causes must be considered (Box 2). Parents may become overwhelmed and frustrated with a constantly crying young infant; look for signs that a parent is not coping before it becomes a child abuse case. This diagnosis occurs early in life; a suddenly irritable or poorly feeding 8-week-old who was previously healthy is less likely to have colic.

Treatment

There are no medications or treatments that have proven to be very effective and yet safe. Anticholinergic medications work but have too many side effects, such as seizures, respiratory trouble, syncope, and coma; therefore, they are not recommended. Simethicone has not been found to reduce colic. Switching to soy- or whey-based formulas has not been proven definitely to work [77]. Techniques such as swaddling the infant, using a pacifier or the rocking motion of car ride, or placing the infant in a car seat on top of a moving clothes dryer (watch car seat does not fall off dryer) also may work to calm the infant. Reassuring parents that episodes of colic will pass is the best antidote. Encourage parents to allow themselves "time outs" from the child, allowing someone else they trust to care for the child during a crying episode.

Box 2. The inconsolable, crying young infant

Anal fissures
Corneal abrasions
Diaper pins
Formula intolerance
Fractures
Hair tourniquets
Hematoma
Hernias
Infections (eg, UTI or meningitis)
Intussusception
Otitis media
Reactions to medications such as decongestants

Hypertrophic pyloric stenosis

Pathophysiology

Hypertrophic pyloric stenosis (HPS) is a narrowing of the pyloric canal caused by hypertrophy of the musculature. The cause of this condition remains unclear, but some experts theorize that HPS is caused by *Helicobacter pylori*, the same bacteria associated with peptic ulcer disease. This theory is based on nonspecific evidence, such as the temporal distribution, seasonality, and familial clustering of HPS, along with the pathologic finding of leukocytic infiltrates, and the increased incidence seen in association with bottle-feeding [78].

Causes

HPS occurs in 1 of every 250 births and appears predominantly in males (male to female ratio of 4:1). The condition also has racial variation. It is observed to be more common in whites than in African Americans and is rare in Asians. Originally, first-born males were believed to be affected more often, but it is now known that birth order is not a factor. A child of an affected parent has an increased chance of HPS, with the risk being higher if the mother was affected [79].

Presentation

HPS usually presents during the third to fifth week of life. Symptoms begin rather benignly, with occasional vomiting at the end of feeding or soon thereafter. This is when HPS is often confused with a viral syndrome, gastroesophageal (GE) reflux, or milk intolerance. Emesis is nonbilious because the stenosis is proximal to the duodenum. As the disease progresses, the incidence of vomiting increases, now following every feed, and can become projectile. Comparing birth weight to current weight is a key element in the evaluation of a neonate with vomiting. After the first week, healthy neonates should gain approximately 20 to 30 g (1 ounce) per day. Healthy normal infants who "spit up" (regurgitate) will continue to gain weight and grow well. Infants with HPS will continue to be hungry but, because of repeated vomiting, may reach a plateau or even lose weight. An infant with HPS may also become constipated as the result of dehydration and decreased intake.

On examination, the neonate with HPS may appear normal but hungry, or the may have signs of dehydration. Dehydration may lead to the appearance of jaundice. Peristaltic waves moving from left to right may be seen in the left upper quadrant after feeding. A palpable "olive" or small mass in the right upper or middle quadrant, at the lateral margin of the right rectus muscle just below the liver edge, may also be detected during physical examination. Decompressing the stomach with a nasogastric tube first and using a lubricant on the fingertips may improve the ability to palpate this "olive." Clinicians' ability to palpate the pyloric "olive" has decreased over the years, probably because of the addition of ultrasonography in confirming the diagnosis. In 1999, Abbas and colleagues [80] reported that many infants with HPS who have palpable masses on examination still undergo one or more unnecessary and redundant tests. This situation is associated with a delay in diagnosis, increased costs, and possibly adverse clinical health problems.

Differential diagnosis

The differential diagnosis for a vomiting neonate includes the life-threatening disorder of volvulus with or without associated malrotation of the intestine. Infants with volvulus deteriorate rapidly, and the vomiting will be bilious, eventually with signs of sepsis and bowel necrosis. Incarcerated hernias also can present similarly, as well as intussusception (although less commonly in the neonatal period). Viral gastroenteritis can occur in the neonate, but caution is advised when making this diagnosis in infants less than 6 weeks old. At a minimum, significant diarrhea and the presence of ill contacts should both be present before considering viral gastroenteritis.

GE reflux is much more common than pyloric stenosis, and vomiting in the neonatal period is often attributed to GE reflux when other diagnoses should be considered. Vomiting caused by GE reflux usually occurs during feeds or immediately afterwards. The amount of vomitus is smaller, and the neonate will continue to gain weight. Infections, especially in the urinary tract, also can present with vomiting as a chief complaint and an examination of the genitalia and urine is imperative in any infant who presents with vomiting.

Laboratory tests

Prolonged vomiting in HPS causes the infant to lose large quantities of gastric secretions rich in H^+ and Cl^- ions. As a result of dehydration, the kidney attempts to conserve Na^+ ions by exchanging them for K^+ ions. The net result is a loss of both H^+ and K^+ ions. Therefore, the infant with HPS will initially demonstrate a hypokalemic, hypochloremic, metabolic alkalosis [81]. If the infant remains dehydrated for a long period, this alkalosis may eventually turn to acidosis.

Imaging studies

If no small mass or "olive" is palpable in the right upper or middle quadrant of a young infant with a clinical picture suggestive of HPS, further studies are warranted. Ultrasonography measures the thickness of the pyloric wall (normally ≤ 2.0 mm but in HPS is ≥ 4.0 mm) and the length of the pyloric canal (normally ≤ 10.0 mm but in HPS is ≥ 14–16 mm), leading to a diagnosis of HPS. Ultrasonography has been shown to have a sensitivity and specificity as high as 100% [82,83]. A false-negative result may occur if the ultrasonographer measures through the distal stomach or antrum and not through the pylorus itself. A false-positive results if pyloric spasm is present and not pyloric stenosis.

If ultrasonography is nondiagnostic and HPS remains a concern, the next radiologic test of choice is an upper-GI series. The upper GI will show the classic "string sign" as contrast flows through the narrowed pyloric lumen. There will also be delayed gastric emptying. As with ultrasonography, false-positive results may occur because of pyloric spasm, which also gives the appearance of a string sign. Endoscopy also can be used to diagnose HPS but is not used commonly [84].

Management

Once HPS has been diagnosed, admission to the hospital is indicated. Often these infants are dehydrated and therefore hydration and correction of any electrolyte abnormalities should be started in the ED. The surgical procedure required to correct the stenosis is the Ramstedt procedure, which involves incising and separating the hypertrophic muscle fibers of the pylorus.

In Japan, intravenous atropine has been used to decrease the spasm of the pylorus as an alternative to surgery. It is then administered orally for several weeks until the child "outgrows" the stenosis. Surgery has been avoided in many cases [85]; however, surgery remains the standard treatment in the United States.

Malrotation with midgut volvulus

Pathophysiology

Congenital malrotation of the midgut portion of the intestine is often the cause of volvulus in the neonatal period. Malrotation occurs during the fifth to eighth week in embryonic life when the intestine projects out of the abdominal cavity, rotates 270°, and then returns into the abdomen. If the rotation is not correct, the intestine will not be "fixed down" correctly at the mesentery, and the vascular mesentery will appear more stalk-like in its structure and is at risk later for twisting, called volvulus. Volvulus is the twisting of a loop of bowel about its mesenteric base stalk attachment; ischemia subsequently develops, and this constitutes a true surgical emergency because bowel necrosis can occur within hours. The entire small bowel is at risk for ischemia and necrosis.

Causes

The incidence of volvulus peaks during the first month of life but can present anytime in childhood. The male to female ratio is 2:1, and this is rarely a familial disorder. The exact frequency of midgut volvulus is not known because it is frequently asymptomatic. Congenital adhesions, called Ladd's bands, extending from the cecum to the liver, are associated with congenital malrotation. These adhesions may cause external compression of the duodenum and obstruction. This condition is not generally considered a surgical emergency, but it eventually requires surgical intervention to lyse these bands.

Presentation

Volvulus may present in one of three ways: (1) as a sudden onset of bilious vomiting and abdominal pain in a neonate; (2) as a history of "feeding problems" with bilious vomiting that now appears like a bowel obstruction; and (3) although less commonly, as a failure to thrive with severe feeding intolerance [86]. Bilious vomiting in a neonate is always worrisome and is a surgical emergency until proven otherwise. If the bowel is already ischemic or necrotic, the neonate may present with a pale complexion and grunting. The abdomen may or may not be distended depending on the location of the volvulus. If the obstruction is proximal, there may be no distension. The abdominal wall may appear "blue" if the bowel is already ischemic or necrotic. The pain is constant, not intermittent, and the neonate will appear irritable. Jaundice also may be present. Hematochezia is a late sign and indicates intestinal necrosis. Neonates who have volvulus will gradually deteriorate if bowel remains ischemic.

Differential diagnosis

As stated earlier, bilious vomiting in a neonate is considered a surgical emergency until proven otherwise. However, in the early presentation of volvulus, vomitus may be nonbilious, and a misdiagnosis of acute gastroenteritis may result. As in the discussion of pyloric stenosis, the acute gastroenteritis should be diagnosed cautiously in young infants. In pyloric stenosis, vomitus is always nonbilious. The duration of symptoms with pyloric stenosis is usually longer, and the child usually appears well, although possibly dehydrated and hungry. Incarcerated hernias may also present with bilious vomiting. It is therefore imperative to thoroughly examine a vomiting neonate for signs of a hernia. Rarer causes of bilious vomiting include duodenal or ileal atresia, although this is discovered typically in the newborn nursery or soon after. With intestinal atresia, the neonate will not be as ill appearing as with volvulus. Necrotizing enterocolitis also can rarely appear in term neonates. Intestinal hematomas may occur in cases of child abuse.

Congenital adrenal hyperplasia (CAH) can cause bilious vomiting without anatomical obstruction. It may present in the first few weeks of life. CAH results in adrenal insufficiency with decreased cortisol levels and salt wasting. Infants will present with hypotension and electrolyte imbalance (low Na^+ and high K^+). It is more likely that CAH will be seen in male infants who present in the ED. Female newborns who have this condition are less commonly missed in the newborn nursery because the accumulation of androgenic compounds affects the external genitalia to a greater extent. Hirschsprung's disease or congenital intestinal aganglionosis also may also present with bilious vomiting. In this condition, there should also be a history of decreased stool output since birth.

Laboratory tests

Laboratory tests are nonspecific for volvulus. Typically, blood tests will show signs of dehydration and acidosis.

Diagnostic imaging

The classic finding on abdominal plain films is the "double bubble sign," which shows a paucity of gas (airless abdomen) with two air bubbles, one in the stomach, and one in the duodenum (Fig. 1). Other findings may include air–fluid levels, a paucity of gas distally, or dilated loops over the liver shadow. The plain film also can be entirely normal.

An upper-GI contrast study is considered the gold standard for diagnosing volvulus. The classic finding is that of the small intestine rotated to the right side of the abdomen (an indication of the malrotation), with contrast narrowing at the site of obstruction, causing a "cork-screwing" appearance. Air as a contrast agent has recently gained more acceptance for the diagnosis of high-GI obstructions such as volvulus and low-GI obstructions such as intussusception [87]. Ultrasonography also has been studied for diagnosing volvulus. The ultrasonography may show a distended, fluid-filled duodenum, increased peritoneal fluid, and dilated small bowel loops to the right of the spine [88,89]. Sometimes, spiraling of the small bowel around the superior mesenteric artery also can be observed [90].

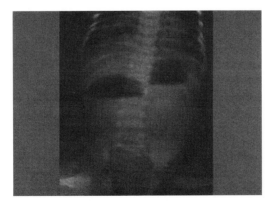

Fig. 1. The classic finding of malrotation with midgut volvulus on abdominal plain films is the "double bubble sign," which shows a paucity of gas (airless abdomen) with two air bubbles, one in the stomach and one in the duodenum.

Management

Because of the risk of bowel necrosis and resulting sepsis, diagnosing this life-threatening condition as early as possible is imperative. Once malrotation with midgut volvulus has been diagnosed, aggressive resuscitation using boluses of normal saline, 20 cc/kg, and the placement of a nasogastric tube should occur. Antibiotics should be administered to cover gram-positive, gram-negative, and anaerobic flora (eg, ampicillin, gentamicin, and clindamycin). Consultation with a pediatric surgeon should not be delayed for diagnostic studies. The sooner the child is admitted to the operating room, the lower the morbidity and mortality of this condition. Some pediatric surgeons will take an ill-appearing neonate with bilious vomiting directly to the operating room without any additional diagnostic tests.

Necrotizing enterocolitis

Causes

Necrotizing enterocolitis (NEC) is seen typically in the neonatal intensive care unit, occurring in premature infants in their first few weeks of life. Occasionally, it is encountered in the term infant, usually within the first 10 days after birth. The cause of NEC is unknown, but a history of an anoxic episode at birth and other neonatal stressors are associated with the diagnosis [91,92].

Pathophysiology

The pathologic finding of NEC is that of a necrotic segment of bowel with gas accumulation in the submucosa. Necrosis can lead to perforation, sepsis, and death. The distal ileum and proximal colon are most commonly involved. *Clostridium* spp, *E coli*, *Staphylococcus epidermidis*, and rotavirus are the pathogens recovered most commonly [72,73].

Presentation

Infants who have NEC will present typically as appearing quite ill, with lethargy, irritability, decreased oral intake, distended abdomen, and bloody stools. Symptoms may present in a range from fairly mild, with only occult-blood positive stools, to a much more critically ill presentation. Because this condition is diagnosed typically in the neonatal intensive care unit, it still must be considered in a term infant who has experienced significant stress, such as anoxia, at birth.

Radiologic studies

The plain abdominal film finding of pneumatosis intestinalis, caused by gas in the intestinal wall, is diagnostic of NEC.

Management

Management includes fluid resuscitation, bowel rest, and broad-spectrum antibiotic coverage. Early surgical consultation is imperative.

Summary

Abdominal pain or gastrointestinal symptoms are common complaints in young children. It is the emergency physician's duty to understand current recommendations regarding the evaluation and management of more benign conditions such as gastroenteritis and also be able to differentiate a true surgical condition such as appendicitis.

References

[1] Kim M, Strait RT, Sato TT, et al. A randomized clinical trial of analgesia in children with acute abdominal pain. Acad Emerg Med 2002;9(4):281–7.

[2] Gorelick M. Validity and reliability of clinical signs in the diagnosis of dehydration in children. Pediatrics 1997;99(5):e6.

[3] Duggan C, Refat M, Hashem M, et al. How valid are clinical signs of dehydration in infants? J Pediatr Gastroenterol Nutr 1996;22:56–61.

[4] Lee PH, Bank DE, Flomenbaum N. Hypoglycemia and ABC's (sugar). Ann Emerg Med 2000; 36(3):278–9.

[5] Atherly-John YC, Cunningham SJ, Crain EF. A randomized trial of oral vs intravenous rehydration in a pediatric emergency department. Arch Peds Adol Med 2002;156:1240–3.

[6] Nager A, Wang VJ. Comparison of nasogastric and intravenous methods of rehydration in pediatric patients with acute dehydration. Pediatrics 2002;109(4):566–72.

[7] American Academy of Pediatrics. Subcommittee on Acute Gastroenteritis Practice parameter: the management of acute gastroenteritis in young children. Pediatrics 1996;97(3):424–35.

[8] Reeves J, Shannon M, Fleisher G. Ondansetron decreases vomiting associated with acute gastroenteritis: a randomized, controlled trial. Pediatrics 2002;109(4):e62.

[9] Ramsook C, Sahagun-Carreon L, Kozinetz C, et al. A randomized clinical trial comparing ondansetron with placebo in children with vomiting from acute gastroenteritis. Ann Emerg Med 2002;39(4):397–403.

[10] Van Niel CW, Feudtner C, Garrison MM, et al. Meta-analysis of *Lactobacillus* therapy. Pediatrics 2002;109:678–84.

[11] Tolia V, Lin CH, Elitsur Y. A prospective randomized study with mineral oil and oral lavage solution for treatment of faecal impaction in children. Aliment Pharmacol Ther 1993;7: 523–9.

[12] Bishop WP. Miracle laxative? J Pediatr Gastroenterol Nutr 2001;32:514–5.

[13] Reedy J, Zwiren J. Enema-induced hypocalcemia and hyperphosphatemia leading to cardiac arrest during induction of anesthesia in an outpatient surgery center. Anesthesiology 1983; 59:578.

[14] Ziskind A, Gellis SS. Water intoxication following tap water enemas. AMA J Dis Child 1958; 96:699–704.

[15] Wagner JM, McKinner WP, Carpenter JL. Does this patient have appendicitis? JAMA 1996; 276(19):1589–94.

[16] Williams A, Bello M. Perforation rates relates to delayed presentation in childhood acute appendicitis. J R Coll Surg Edinb 1998;43:101–2.

[17] Saidi RF, Ghasemi M. Role of Alvarado score in diagnosis and treatment of suspected acute appendicitis. Am J Emerg Med 2000;18(2):230–1.

[18] Horwitz JR, Gursoy M, Jaksic T, et al. Importance of diarrhea as a presenting symptom of appendicitis in very young children. Am J Surg 1997;173(2):80–2.

[19] Scholer SJ, Pituch K, Orr DP, et al. Use of the rectal examination on children with acute abdominal pain. Pediatr Clin N Am 1998;37(5):311–6.

[20] Rothrock SG, Pagane J. Acute appendicitis in children: emergency department diagnosis and management. Ann Emerg Med 2000;36(1):39–51.

[21] Emery M, Jones J, Brown M. Clinical application of infrared thermography in the diagnosis of appendicitis. Am J Emerg Med 1994;42(1):48–50.

[22] Reynolds SL. Missed appendicitis in a pediatric emergency department. Pediatr Emerg Care 1993;9(1):1–3.

[23] Coleman C, Thompson JE, Bennion RS, et al. White blood cell count is poor predictor of severity of disease in the diagnosis of appendicitis. Am Surg 1998;64(10):983–5.

[24] Chung JL, Kong MS, Lin SL, et al. Diagnostic value of C-reactive protein in children with perforated appendicitis. Eur J Pediatr 1996;155(7):529–31.

[25] Paajanen H, Mansikka A, Laato M, et al. Are serum inflammatory markers age dependent in acute appendicitis? J Am Coll Surg 1997;184(3):303–8.

[26] Hallan S, Asberg A, Edna TH. Additional value of biochemical tests in suspected acute appendicitis. Eur J Surg 1997;163(7):533–8.

[27] Andersson RE, Hugander AP, Ghazi SH, et al. Diagnostic value of disease history, clinical presentation, and inflammatory parameters in appendicitis. World J Surg 1999;23(2):133–40.

[28] Albiston E. The role of radiological imaging in the diagnosis of acute appendicitis. Can J Gastroenterol 2002;16(7):451–63.

[29] Orr RK, Porter D, Hartman D. Ultrasonography to evaluate adults for appendicitis: decision making based on meta-analysis and probabilistic reasoning. Acad Emerg Med 1995;2(7):644–50.

[30] Wong ML, Casey SO, Leonidas JC, et al. Sonographic diagnosis of acute appendicitis in children. J Pediatr Surg 1994;29(10):1356–60.

[31] Ramachandran P, Sivit CJ, Newman KD, et al. Ultrasonography as an adjunct in the diagnosis of acute appendicitis: a 4-year experience. J Pediatr Surg 1996;31(1):164–7 [disussion: 167–9].

[32] Crady SK, Jones JS, Wyn T, et al. Clinical validity of ultrasound in children with suspected appendicitis. Ann Emerg Med 1993;22(7):1125–9.

[33] Zaki AM, MacMahon RA, Gray AR. Acute appendicitis in children: when does ultrasound help? Aust N Z J Surg 1994;64(10):695–8.

[34] Hahn HB, Hoepner FU, Kalle T, et al. Sonography of acute appendicitis in children: 7 years experience. Pediatr Radiol 1998;28(3):147–51.

[35] Carrico CW, Fenton LZ, Taylor GA, et al. Impact of sonography on the diagnosis and treatment of acute lower abdominal pain in children and young adults. Am J Roentgenol 1999;172(2):513–6.

[36] Lessin MS, Chan M, Catallozzi M, et al. Selective use of ultrasonography for acute appendicitis in children. Am J Surg 1999;177(3):193–6.

[37] Rice HE, Arbesman M, Martin DJ, et al. Does early ultrasonography affect management of pediatric appendicitis? a prospective analysis. J Pediatr Surg 1999;34(5):754–9.

[38] Rice HE, Arbesman M, Martin DJ, et al. Does early ultrasonography affect management of pediatric appendicitis? a prospective analysis. J Pediatr Surg 1999;34(5):754–9 [discussion: 758–9].

[39] Roosevelt GE, Reynolds SL. Does the use of ultrasonography improve the outcome of children with appendicitis? Acad Emerg Med 1998;5(11):1071–5.

[40] Quillin SP, Siegel MJ. Diagnosis of appendiceal abscess in children with acute appendicitis: value of color Doppler sonography. Am J Roentgenol 1995;164(5):1251–4.

[41] Funaki B, Grosskreutz SR, Funaki CN. Using unenhanced helical CT with enteric contrast material for suspected appendicitis in patients treated at a community hospital. Am J Roentgenol 1998;171(4):997–1001.
[42] Garcia Pena BM, Mandl KD, Kraus SJ, et al. Ultrasonography and limited computed tomography in the diagnosis and management of appendicitis in children. JAMA 1999;282(11): 1041–6.
[43] Pena BM, Taylor GA, Lund DP, et al. Effect of computed tomography on patient management and costs in children with suspected appendicitis. Pediatrics 1999;104(3 Pt 1):440–6.
[44] Rao PM, Rhea JT, Rattner DW. Introduction of appendiceal CT: impact on negative appendectomy and appendiceal perforation rates. Ann Surg 1999;229(3):344–9.
[45] Jabra AA, Shalaby-Rana EI, Fishman EK. CT of appendicitis in children. J Comput Assist Tomogr 1997;21(4):661–6.
[46] Kanegaye JT, Vance CW, Parisi M, et al. Failure of technetium-99m hexamethylpropylene amine oxime leukocyte scintigraphy in the evaluation of children with suspected appendicitis. Ped Emerg Care 1995;11(5):285–90.
[47] Turan C, Tutus A, Ozokutan BH, et al. The evaluation of technetium 99m-citrate scintigraphy in children with suspected appendicitis. J Pediatr Surg 1999;34(8):1272–5.
[48] Hormann M, Paya K, Eibenberger K, et al. MR imaging in children with nonperforated acute appendicitis: value of unenhanced MR imaging in sonographically selected cases. Am J Roentgenol 1998;171(2):467–70.
[49] Banani SA, Talei A. Can oral metronidazole substitute parenteral drug therapy in acute appendicitis? a new policy in the management of simple or complicated appendicitis with localized peritonitis: a randomized controlled clinical trial. Am Surg 1999;65(5):411–6.
[50] Soderquist-Elinder C, Hirsch K, Bergdahl S, et al. Prophylactic antibiotics in uncomplicated appendicitis during childhood–a prospective randomised study. Eur J Pediatr Surg 1995;5(5): 282–5.
[51] Parashar UD, Holman RC, Cummings KD, et al. Trends in intussusception-associated hospitalizations and deaths among US infants. Pediatrics 2000;106(6):1413–21.
[52] Ugwu BT, Legbo JN, Dakum NK, et al. Childhood intussusception: a 9-year review. Ann Trop Paediatr 2000;20(2):131–5.
[53] Kuppermann N, O'Dea T, Pinckney L, et al. Predictors of intussusception in young children. Arch Pediatr Adolesc Med 2000;154(3):250–5.
[54] Heldrich FJ. Lethargy as a presenting symptom in patients with intussusception. Clin Pediatr 1986;25(7):363–5.
[55] Yamamoto LG, Morita SY, Boychuk R, et al. Stool appearance in intussusception: assessing the value of the term "currant jelly." Am J Emerg Med 1997;15(3):293–8.
[56] Smith DS, Bonadio WA, Losek JD, et al. The role of abdominal x-rays in the diagnosis and management of intussusception. Pediatr Emerg Care 1992;8(6):325–7.
[57] Yang ST, Tsai CH, Chen JA, et al. Differential diagnosis between intussusception and gastroenteritis by plain film. Acta Paediatr Taiwan 1995;36(3):170–5.
[58] Bhisitkul DM, Listernick R, Shkolnik A, et al. Clinical application of ultrasonography in the diagnosis of intussusception. J Pediatr 1992;121(2):182–6.
[59] Campbell JB. Contrast media in intussusception. Pediatr Radiol 1989;19(5):293–6.
[60] Gonzalez-Spinola J, Del Pozo G, Tejedor D, et al. Intussusception: the accuracy of ultrasound-guided saline enema and the usefulness of a delayed attempt at reduction. J Pediatr Surg 1999; 34(6):1016–20.
[61] Rohrschneider WK, Troger J. Hydrostatic reduction of intussusception under US guidance. Pediatr Radiol 1995;25(7):530–4.
[62] Wang G, Liu XG, Zitsman JL. Nonfluoroscopic reduction of intussusception by air enema. World J Surg 1995;19(3):435–8.
[63] Daneman A, Alton DJ, Ein S, et al. Perforation during attempted intussusception reduction in children: a comparison of perforation with barium and air. Pediatr Radiol 1995;25(2): 81–8.

[64] Gu L, Alton DJ, Daneman A, et al. John Caffey Award: intussusception reduction in children by rectal insufflation of air. Am J Roentgenol 1988;150(6):1345–8.
[65] Schmit P, Rohrschneider WK, Christmann D. Intestinal intussusception survey about diagnostic and nonsurgical therapeutic procedures. Pediatr Radiol 1999;29(10):752–61.
[66] Sandler AD, Ein SH, Connolly B. Unsuccessful air-enema reduction of intussusception: is a second attempt worthwhile? Pediatr Surg Int 1999;15(3–4):214–6.
[67] Lui KW, Wong HF, Cheung YC, et al. Air enema for diagnosis and reduction of intussusception in children: clinical experience and fluoroscopy time correlation. J Pediatr Surg 2001; 36(3):479–81.
[68] Guo JZ, Ma XY, Zhou QH. Results of air pressure enema reduction of intussusception: 6,396 cases in 13 years. J Pediatr Surg 1986;21(12):1201–3.
[69] Kornecki A, Daneman A, Navarro O, et al. Spontaneous reduction of intussusception: clinical spectrum, management and outcome. Pediatr Radiol 2000;30(1):58–63.
[70] Vicario S, Price T. Intestinal obstruction. In: Tintinelli J, Kelen G, Stapczynski J, editors. Emergency medicine: a comprehensive study guide. New York: McGraw-Hill; 2000. p. 539–43.
[71] Brolin RE, Krasna MJ, Mast B. Use of tubes and radiographs in bowel obstruction. Ann Surg 1987;206:126.
[72] Kusamoto H, Yoshida M, Takahashi I, et al. Complications and diagnosis of Meckel's diverticulum in 776 patients. Am J Surg 1992;164:382.
[73] Murali VP, Divaker D, Thachil MV, et al. Meckel's diverticulum in adults. J Indian Med Assoc 1989;87:116.
[74] Wyllie R. Intestinal duplications, meckel diverticulum, and other remnants of the omphalomesentric duct. In: Behrman R, Kliegman R, Jenson H, editors. Nelson textbook of pediatrics. 17th edition. Philadelphia: Elsevier; 2004. p. 1236–7.
[75] Hostetler M, Bracikowski A. Pediatric gastrointestinal disorders. In: Marx J, Hockberger R, Walls R, editors. Rosen's emergency medicine concepts and clinical practice. 5th edition. St Louis (MO): Mosby; 2002. p. 2296–314.
[76] St-Vil D, Brandt ML, Panic S, et al. Meckel's diverticulum in children: a 20 year review. J Pediatr Surg 1991;26(11):1289–92.
[77] Wade S. "Infantile colic": review of therapeutic trials for colic. BMJ 2001;323:437–40.
[78] Paulozzi LJ. Is Helicobacter pylori a cause of infantile hypertrophic pyloric stenosis? Med Hypotheses 2000;55(2):119–25.
[79] Spicer RD. Infantile hypertrophic pyloric stenosis: a review. Br J Surg 1982;69(3):128–35.
[80] Abbas AE, Weiss SM, Alvear DT. Infantile hypertrophic pyloric stenosis: delays in diagnosis and overutilization of imaging modalities. Am Surg 1999;65(1):73–6.
[81] Smith GA, Mihalov L, Shields BJ. Diagnostic aids in the differentiation of pyloric stenosis from severe gastroesophageal reflux during early infancy: the utility of serum bicarbonate and serum chloride. Am J Emerg Med 1999;17(1):28–31.
[82] Hernanz-Schulman M, Sells LL, Ambrosino MM, et al. Hypertrophic pyloric stenosis in the infant without a palpable olive: accuracy of sonographic diagnosis. Radiology 1994;193(3): 771–6.
[83] Neilson D, Hollman AS. The ultrasonic diagnosis of infantile hypertrophic pyloric stenosis: technique and accuracy. Clin Radiol 1994;49(4):246–7.
[84] De Backer A, Bove T, Vandenplas Y, et al. Contribution of endoscopy to early diagnosis of hypertrophic pyloric stenosis. J Pediatr Gastroenterol Nutr 1994;18(1):78–81.
[85] Yamamoto A, Kino M, Sasaki T, et al. Ultrasonographic follow-up of the healing process of medically treated hypertrophic pyloric stenosis. Pediatr Radiol 1998;28(3):177–8.
[86] Lin JN, Lou CC, Wang KL. Intestinal malrotation and midgut volvulus: a 15-year review. J Formos Med Assoc 1995;94(4):178–81.
[87] Harrison RL, Set P, Brain AJ. Persistent value of air-augmented radiograph in neonatal high gastrointestinal obstruction, despite more modern techniques. Acta Paediatr 1999;88(11): 1284–6.
[88] Shimanuki Y, Aihara T, Takano H, et al. Clockwise whirlpool sign at color Doppler US: an objective and definite sign of midgut volvulus. Radiology 1996;199(1):261–4.

[89] Weinberger E, Winters WD, Liddell RM, et al. Sonographic diagnosis of intestinal malrotation in infants: importance of the relative positions of the superior mesenteric vein and artery. Am J Roentgenol 1992;159(4):825–8.
[90] Zerin JM, DiPietro MA. Superior mesenteric vascular anatomy at ultrasound in patients with surgically proved malrotation of the midgut. Radiology 1992;183(3):693–4.
[91] Kliegman R, Walsh M. Neonatal necrotizing enterocolitis: pathogenesis, classification, and spectrum of illness. Curr Probl Pediatr 1987;27:215.
[92] Kulkarni A, Vigneswaran R. Necrotizing enterocolitis. Indian J Pediatr 2001;68(9):847–53.

ELSEVIER
SAUNDERS

Pediatr Clin N Am 53 (2006) 139–155

PEDIATRIC CLINICS

OF NORTH AMERICA

Emergency Medical Treatment and Labor Act: The Basics and Other Medicolegal Concerns

Getachew Teshome, MD*, Forrest T. Closson, MD

*Department of Pediatrics, Division of Emergency Medicine,
University of Maryland Hospital for Children, 22 South Greene Street, Baltimore, MD 21201, USA*

The Emergency Medical Treatment and Labor Act (EMTALA), also known as the "patient antidumping" statute was passed in 1986 as part of the Consolidated Omnibus Budget Reconciliation Act of 1985 (COBRA). Congress enacted these provisions because of its concern with an "increasing number of reports" that hospital emergency rooms were refusing to accept or treat individuals with emergency conditions if the individuals did not have insurance [1].

The statute is not the first attempt by the government to ensure access to emergency care. In 1946, Congress passed public law 79–725, the Hospital Survey and Construction Act, sponsored by Senators Lister Hill and Harold Burton, widely known as the Hill-Burton Act. It was the nation's major health facility construction program under Title VI of the Public Health Service Act. Originally designed to provide Federal grants to modernize hospitals that had become obsolete because of a lack of capital investment throughout the period of the Great Depression and World War II (1929 to 1945), the program has changed over time to address other types of needs. In return for Federal funds, facilities agreed to provide free or reduced charge medical services to persons unable to pay. In 1970, direct loans and loan guarantees with interest subsidies to facilities were authorized, and in 1972, a 20-year limit on the provision of uncompensated services and specific requirements for providing uncompensated services was initiated [2].

In 1975, Congress enacted Title XVI of the Public Health Service Act, an amendment to the Hill-Burton act. Facilities assisted under Title XVI were required to provide uncompensated services in perpetuity. The same title trans-

---

* Corresponding author.
  E-mail address: Gteshome@peds.umaryland.edu (G. Teshome).

ferred the enforcement responsibilities from the states to the Federal government and required more stringent investigation, monitoring, and compliance standards [3,4].

Despite the above regulations, unstable patients were being transferred or denied care simply because they did not have the financial means to make or guarantee hospital payment. In response, the US Congress enacted legislation entitled the Emergency Medical Treatment and Active Labor Act (EMTALA), in 1986 [5]. The Act is tailored to prevent injury to patients arising from economically based treatment delays and to guarantee access to emergency medical services without regard to economic status.

Definition of EMTALA

"If an individual. . .comes to the emergency department and a request is made on the individual's behalf for examination or treatment for a medical condition, the hospital must provide for an appropriate medical screening examination within the capability of the hospital's emergency department, including ancillary services routinely available to the emergency department, to determine whether or not an emergency medical condition. . .exists" [5].

If the individual has an emergency medical condition, the hospital must provide either "within the staff and facilities available at the hospital, for such further medical examination and such treatment as may be required to stabilize the medical condition, or transfer the individual to another facility" [5].

Neither the screening examination nor any necessary stabilizing treatment may be delayed to inquire into the patient's method of payment or insurance status. If a hospital fails to meet these obligations, it is subject to a civil monetary penalty of up to $50,000 per violation and may have its Medicare provider agreement terminated by the Secretary of the US Department of Health and Human Services (HHS). In certain circumstances, a hospital may also be fined for its failure to accept an appropriate transfer if it has the staff and equipment to treat the patient. Physicians who negligently violate the law are also subject to a civil monetary penalty of up to $50,000 for each violation and may be excluded from participating in the Medicare and Medicaid programs for repeated violations or for even a single violation that is gross and flagrant [5].

Hospitals and medical professionals have charged repeatedly that EMTALA obligations are burdensome, complex, inefficient, and unclear. There are ambiguities in the language of the act and they lack specific definitions. To help promote the consistent application of the regulations concerning the special responsibilities of Medicare-participating hospitals in emergency cases, on September 9, 2003, the Department of Health and Human Services, Centers for Medicare and Medicaid Services (CMS) published "Clarifying Policies Related to the Responsibilities of Medicare-Participating Hospitals in Treating Individuals With Emergency Medical Conditions (Final Regulations)" [1].

Unchanged regulations

1. Hospitals are still required to report receipt of unstabilized patient transferred without a certification from a physician that the benefits of transfer exceed the risks and if a patient comes to the emergency department saying he went to another hospital's emergency department and was refused service because he had no proof of insurance.
2. Hospitals still must post signs in the emergency department describing patients' EMTALA rights.
3. Hospitals must maintain patient records, physician on-call lists, and emergency department logs.
4. Hospitals with "specialized capabilities" cannot refuse to accept the transfer of a patient needing those specialized capabilities, subject to certain specific limitations, also known as "reverse dumping."

The new changes

1. The EMTALA does not apply to patients after they have been admitted to the hospital, including admitted patients who are boarded in the emergency department.
2. The scope of hospital property (and the phrase "comes to the emergency department") is more narrowly tailored.
3. The EMTALA no longer applies to hospital owned and operated ambulance services that follow local or state EMS protocols for diversion.
4. Requirements for physicians serving on hospital on-call panels have been relaxed.
5. The EMTALA allows hospitals to follow reasonable registration procedures in the emergency department as long as the procedures do not result in a delay in performing the screening examination or treatment [1].

Potential ambiguities in the interpretation of the act

To be a dedicated emergency department (ED), the department must either:

A. Be licensed by the state as an emergency department (applicable in states that license emergency departments separately from hospitals),
B. Be offered to the public as an emergency department or urgent care center, or
C. Have provided one third of its visits on an urgent basis without requiring a previously scheduled appointment in the previous year [6].

Appropriate medical screening examination

An examination must be provided within the capability of the hospital's emergency department to determine whether or not an emergency medical condition exists. An appropriate medical screening must be performed by a physician or "qualified medical personnel" (QMP). A QMP is a coined term only in the context of EMTALA and refers to a practitioner who has been approved by the medical staff and is endorsed according to the Medical Staff Bylaws or the Medical Staff Rules and Regulations [7].

Emergency medical condition

A medical condition manifesting itself by acute symptoms of sufficient severity, including severe pain, psychiatric disturbances, or symptoms of substance abuse, such that the absence of immediate medical attention could reasonably be expected to result in (a) placing the health of the individual in serious jeopardy; (b) serious impairment to bodily functions; or (c) serious dysfunction of any bodily organ or part [7,8].

Stabilization

Within reasonable clinical confidence, no material deterioration of the condition is likely to result from or occur during the transfer of the individual from the facility.

Appropriate transfer

1. The transferring hospital has provided medical treatment within its capacity and has deemed that, within reasonable probability, no material deterioration in clinical condition is likely to occur during transportation.
2. The receiving facility has agreed to accept the patient and has the necessary equipment and staff to handle the clinical situation.
3. The transferring facility sends all appropriate medical records with the patient and provides appropriate transportation, or
4. If transferring an unstable patient, the transfer certification must address the following elements:
   a. Patient's condition
   b. Benefits of transfer
   c. Risk of transfer
   d. Specific information regarding the receiving facility, such as names of facility, names of physicians accepting the patient, the facility provided with all necessary medical records and a statement that a patient report was called to the accepting facility
   e. Description of the mode of transportation

f. Patient must sign a consent and certify whether the transfer was initiated on patient request, physician request, or other

g. Form must be witnessed and the patient must sign that he or she understands the risks and benefits of transfer [9,10]

Controversies

Over the last decade physicians have raised multiple concerns about the implementation of EMTALA in their practice. Some of the concerns have been answered by the final regulation published in 2003 by the Department of Health and Human Services, Centers for Medicare and Medicaid Services (CMS), as "Clarifying Policies Related to the Responsibilities of Medicare-Participating Hospitals in Treating Individuals With Emergency Medical Conditions" [1]. The concerns that are still controversial are

1. Did EMTALA contribute to over-crowding of our emergency departments?
2. Are we providing expensive health care in the emergency setting for non-emergent conditions?
3. With an increasing number of uninsured patients, are hospitals forced to see patients without reimbursement?

The most reliable data on ED visits come from the National Hospital Ambulatory Medical Care Survey, which has been conducted annually since 1992 by the National Center for Health Statistics. During the period from 1993 through 2003, the number of ED visits increased by 26%, from 90.3 million annual ED visits in 1993 to 113.9 million annually in 2003. This represents an average increase of more than 2 million visits per year. On the other hand, the number of hospital EDs in the United States decreased by approximately 12.3% during the same period [11]. These and other reports suggest that ED crowding is a reflection of larger supply-and-demand mismatches within the health care system, most notably the lack of surge capacity in our nation's hospitals, coupled with the increasing use of the ED by an uninsured population for routine health care.

The growing uninsured and underinsured population threatens the financial viability of the entire health care delivery system, including the emergency medical services infrastructure. The lack of adequate Medicaid and Medicare funding and payments has served not only to increase the number of patients forced to access the health care system through EDs but also to simultaneously increase the cost of operating EDs. Likewise, the Professional Liability Insurance crisis has served to increase the number of patients accessing the health care system through EDs, because private practices have closed, moved, or have limited their scope of practice; at the same time, the liability insurance costs for emergency medicine have increased dramatically, threatening the viability of individual hospital independent democratic groups [12].

Despite economic expansion, the number of uninsured United States residents has increased. Many uninsured patients use hospital emergency departments as a vital portal of entry to access the health care system [13]. During his administration, President Bill Clinton stated that "When people don't have any health insurance, they still get health care. But they get it when it's too late, when it's too expensive—often from the most expensive place of all, the emergency room" [14]. Care in the emergency departments is traditionally thought of as expensive. Williams [15] has found that "the true costs of non-urgent care in the emergency department are relatively low. The potential savings from a diversion of non-urgent visits to private physician's offices may therefore be much less than is widely believed." Cost savings were also reported in a pediatric emergency department by shifting lower-acuity patients within emergency departments to "fast-track" areas [16]. But for patients who do not qualify for care in a fast-track area, the cost of emergency service could be more significant.

A periodic review of the consequences of EMTALA on the emergency medical services by policy makers, professional organizations such as American College of Emergency Physicians, American Academy of Pediatrics, and physicians will prevent the failure of this well-intentioned act. Furthermore, the expectations of the public must be tempered by the realistic capabilities of the emergency medical system and the objective reality of the situations, such as overcrowding and ambulance diversion, which may be the result of an under-funded, under-resourced medical care delivery system. Most patients are unaware of EMTALA and its mandate that emergency medical care be available to all who request it and are equally ignorant that there are few requirements that this care be funded [12]. By convincing the public of the validity of a given position, it is more likely that they will become a secondary lobbying force for appropriate legislative and regulatory change.

Other medicolegal concerns

Privacy and confidentiality

Respect for a patient's privacy and confidentiality has been a long-standing responsibility of physicians. The Oath of Hippocrates states: "What I may see or hear in the course of the treatment or even outside of the treatment in regard to the life of men, which on no account one must spread abroad, I will keep to myself, holding such things shameful to be spoken approximately" [17]. Even though several modern variations have been adopted to reflect a more industrialized society, the basic premises of do no harm and respect for a patient's privacy remain common themes proclaimed by virtually all past and present physicians.

The idea of respect for privacy and confidentiality continues to be an important concept at the forefront of medicine today. The World Medical Association's Declaration of Geneva states: "I will respect the secrets which are confided in me, even after the patient has died" [18]. The American Medical Association's Principles of Medical Ethics states: "A physician shall respect the rights of patients, colleagues, and other health professionals, and shall safeguard patient confidences and privacy within the constraints of the law." [19]. The Code of Ethics for Emergency Physicians states: "Emergency physicians also have a responsibility to protect the confidentiality of patient information. Sensitive information may only be disclosed when such disclosure is necessary to carry out a stronger conflicting duty, such as a duty to protect an identifiable third party from serious harm or to comply with a just law" [20]. In addition, the Joint Commission on Accreditation of Health care Organizations, the nationally recognized accreditation agency for all hospitals within the United States, has adopted explicit standards with respect to patient privacy and confidentiality, which all hospitals must adhere to [21].

In the United States, several state and federal statutes have established the professional and legal obligations of health care providers to protect patient privacy and confidentiality. One of the first legal cases in the United States to address privacy was De May v Roberts (1881), in which a Michigan court upheld a couple's interest in physical privacy after a physician allowed an "unprofessional young unmarried man" to enter their home and assist in the delivery of the couple's baby [22]. The term privacy can be used to mean several things, but in its most basic form, it refers to the idea of being left alone or the condition of being hidden, whereas the term confidentiality refers to the state of being secret [23]. In addition to the invasion of privacy, courts have found physicians liable for the unauthorized release of medical information through a breech of confidentiality in the physician–patient relationship [22].

As a result of concerns about a patient's medical records and issues of privacy and confidentiality, the HHS created a set of regulations known as the Health Insurance Portability and Accountability Act (HIPAA) Privacy Rule. The 1996 HIPPA and the finalized version, known as the Standards for Privacy of Individually Identifiable Health Information (the HIPAA Privacy Rule) is a set of regulations that require health care providers and institutions to adopt a national set of minimum standards to protect medical record privacy and confidentiality [24]. These regulations address the use and disclosure of individuals' health information (called "protected health information") by the organizations subject to the Privacy Rule (called "covered entities"). Covered entities include health plans, health care clearinghouses, and health care providers who conduct health care transactions electronically. A major goal of the Privacy Rule is to assure that an individual's health information is properly protected, while allowing the flow of health information necessary to promote high quality health care and while protecting the public's health and well being.

Decisions to monitor, restrict, or control access to individual medical records may be evaluated by determining whether those accessing the information are primary or secondary users of protected health information. Primary users are clinicians (physicians, nurses, nursing assistants, therapists, and other allied health professionals) who need access to patient information to provide appropriate health care to the patient. Secondary users of health data include researchers, educators, third-party payers, business administrators, legal representatives, auditors, employers, and public health officials [25]. Although not required by the HIPAA Privacy Rule, a covered entity is permitted to disclose protected health information without an individual's authorization to a primary user in several situations, including but not limited to activities involved in the treatment of an individual such as communication between consultants and transmission of records to other health care providers; health care operations, which includes quality assessment and improvement activities; public health activities such as adverse event tracking and communicable disease reporting; threats to individual or public safety such as suicidal or homicidal ideation and terrorist threats; and law enforcement purposes such as court subpoenas, criminal investigations, and the reporting of certain instances of abuse and neglect [24]. A notable exception to the permitted disclosure list is psychotherapy notes. A covered entity must obtain an individual's authorization to use or disclose psychotherapy notes, unless those notes are being used for purposes of treatment by the covered entity that first originated them and in several special circumstances such as averting a serious and imminent threat to public health or safety [24]. A covered entity must obtain the individual's written authorization for any use or disclosure of protected health information that is not otherwise permitted or required by the Privacy Rule or is requested by a secondary user [22].

Other regulations required by the HIPAA Privacy Rule include a written notice of privacy practices be given to all patients on arrival to a covered entity (physician's office, emergency department, inpatient unit, or other area of patient care) and all covered entities must make attempts to obtain a written acknowledgment from all patients of receipt of the privacy practices notice. In addition, all health care institutions must implement policies and procedures to ensure that disclosures of protected health information are restricted to the "minimum necessary" [24].

For all violations of the HIPAA Privacy Rule, HHS may assess civil monetary penalties on a covered entity of $100 per violation, which may not exceed $25,000 per year for multiple identical violations within a calendar year. Within HHS, the Office for Civil Rights has the responsibility for implementing and enforcing the Privacy Rule with respect to voluntary compliance activities and civil money penalties. Criminal penalties are enforced by the US Department of Justice and include a fine of $50,000 and up to 1 year of imprisonment for the intentional receipt or disclosure of protected health information. The criminal penalties increase to a fine of $100,000 and up to 5 years imprisonment for disclosures under false pretenses a fine of $250,000 and up to 10 years imprisonment if the wrongful conduct involves the intent to profit or cause malice [24].

Concerns about privacy and confidentiality with respect to adolescents create an additional challenge. Several studies have clearly shown that concerns about privacy can prevent adolescent patients from seeking care [26–30]. One such study found that half of adolescent females would stop using family planning clinics if parental notification for contraceptives were made mandatory [31], and another study found that over a third of students who did not seek health care did so at least partially because of "not wanting to tell their parents" [32]. To address the growing concerns about an adolescent's right to private and confidential health care, several organizations, including the American Medical Association, the American Academy of Pediatrics, the American Academy of Family Physicians, the American College of Obstetricians and Gynecologists, and the Society for Adolescent Medicine, have issued statements asserting that confidential reproductive health care should be available to minors [33–37].

Specifically with regard to minors (infants, children, and adolescents), the HIPAA Privacy Rule states that in most cases a parent is the "personal representative" of the child and as such can make decisions about access to a child's medical records. A personal representative is a person legally authorized to make health care decisions on an individual's behalf or to act for a deceased individual or the estate. In certain cases, when a parent is not the personal representative of a child, the Privacy Rule defers to state and other applicable laws (such as military or tribal laws) to determine the rights of parents to access and control the protected health information of their minor children. If the laws do not directly address parental access to the minor's protected health information, a covered entity has the discretion to provide or deny a parent's access to the minor's health information, provided the decision is made by a health care professional in the exercise of professional judgment [24]. Those situations in which a parent is not considered to be an adolescent's personal representative include situations in which a state law allows minors to consent for their own care in the absence of parental notification, when a parent agrees to a confidential relationship between a minor and physician, when a physician has a reasonable belief that a child has been subject to some form of abuse, when a court or other law authorizes someone other than the parent to make treatment decisions for a minor, or when treating the parent as the child's personal representative could endanger the child [38].

In addition to HIPAA regulations, there are several other concerns for physicians treating minors, particularly in an emergency setting. Unlike other units in the hospital, where semiprivate and private rooms offer some semblance of privacy and confidentiality, emergency departments house large numbers of patients who rotate frequently and are often separated solely by glass windows or curtains. Several studies have shown that issues of privacy and confidentiality remain a concern for both physicians as well as the patients they treat [39–44].

Consent of care

An important distinction should be made between privacy and confidentiality, as opposed to consent for treatment. By design, the HIPAA Privacy Rule does not address consent for treatment nor does it preempt or change state or other laws that address consent for treatment. The Rule solely addresses access to an individual's personal health information. As a result, if a minor receives emergency medical care without a parent's consent, the parent can obtain the minor's protected health information, unless state or other applicable laws link consent for care and confidentiality [38]. Generally, parents have the legal authority to make medical decisions on behalf of minors based on the belief that minors do not posses the maturity and judgment to make informed decisions before they reach the age of majority (usually 18 years old), and in most cases, it is the parent who consents for a minor's care. However, there are several circumstances when a minor or someone other than a parent may be allowed to consent for care, and in many instances also act as the personal representative. Several of those situations include medical emergencies, care of the mature minor, emancipated minor status, and laws authorizing minors to consent for their own care [45].

Several states have adopted some form of the "mature minor" rule, which allows minors to consent for services without consulting their parents, if the minor is sufficiently intelligent and mature enough to understand the nature and consequences of a proposed treatment [46]. The age at which a minor may be considered to be mature varies from state to state but generally begins around 14 years old. In addition, virtually all states have acknowledged some degree of "emancipated minor." Each state has its own criteria relating to a minor's ability to become emancipated; however, some of the more common criteria include minors who are married, serving in the armed forces, pregnant, parents, high school graduates, older than a certain age, and self sufficient or are living apart from their parents [47]. In addition to mature and emancipated minors, many states have laws that allow minors to consent directly for specific areas of their health care. Several of the more common kinds of health care for which most states allow minors to consent include contraceptive care, pregnancy-related care, sexually transmitted disease and HIV services, substance abuse treatment, and mental heath care [45]. An area of great debate is the minor's ability to consent for abortion services. Although several states include a minor's ability to receive abortion services with general pregnancy care, many do not. In addition, advocates of parental involvement laws contend that policies that give minors the right to consent to sexual health care impair family values and undermine parental authority [46]. Therefore, it is imperative that clinicians be familiar with the specific laws of the jurisdiction in which they practice.

In some instances, a minor will present for care and does not meet the requirements to either consent for their own care or be their own personal representative. A 1993 American Academy of Pediatrics policy statement noted that "fewer than one third of children live in a two parent family in which only the father works outside the home" [47], and 2002 statistics from the United States Department of Labor found that, in 61% of families, both parents work outside the home and that an estimated 19 million families of children younger than 14 have some form of child care requirement [48]. Because increasing numbers of children are being supervised outside of the family, more children are being brought to the emergency department for treatment without the presence of a legal guardian. One study has found that 2% to 3% of all children seeking treatment in an emergency department were not accompanied by a parent or guardian [49]. Generally, laws have supported health care providers in evaluating and treating children without the consent of a parent or guardian.

According to the EMTALA guidelines, an emergency department has a legal obligation to provide a "medical screening" examination for every patient presenting to an emergency department. As a result, when a minor presents for care but cannot consent for care or act as their own personal representative, it is a mandated duty of the emergency department to provide the minimum service of a medical screening evaluation. If an emergency medical condition is identified, then the emergency department should make reasonable attempts to contact the minor's personal representative to obtain consent for care. In the absence of the personal representative, the emergency department is required to use the prudent layperson standards and professional judgment to determine the level of care given. Appropriate medical care for a minor should never be withheld or delayed because of problems obtaining consent [48]. A comprehensive reference from the American College of Emergency Physicians states: "Thus, under federal law, a minor can be examined, treated, stabilized, and even transferred to another hospital for emergency care without consent ever being obtained from the parent or legal guardian" [50]. If no emergency medical condition is identified, then the minor should be instructed to contact a personal representative to obtain consent for care; however, in at least one major pediatric emergency department "it is the practice to treat all patients who present to [the] ED, even if unaccompanied by a parent or caretaker" [51].

An area of growing concern is the minor who presents for care with a parent or guardian whose judgment is impaired by alcohol or drugs. The Children of Alcoholics Foundation estimates that between 11 and 17 million children in the United States are living currently with an alcoholic parent [52], and it has been estimated that one in four children in the United States are exposed to alcohol abuse or dependence in a family member [53]. The US Department of Health and Human Services estimates that approximately 10% of adults and 3% of adolescents in the United States are addicted to alcohol or other drugs [54]. Although the exact number of adults who abuse illicit or prescription drugs remains unknown, clearly there are a significant number of children who are living in homes with drug-abusing parents. As a result, health care personnel who care for children can reasonably expect to encounter minors who are brought for care by parents whose judgment may be impaired by alcohol and drugs.

As a result of this growing problem, the American Academy of Pediatrics has issued multiple policies regarding consent of care for minors. First, the Academy recognizes that there are several fundamental conditions that must be met in order for a parent or guardian to be able to consent for the care of a minor, including that the right to consent to medical treatment for a minor must be delegated to a legally and medically competent adult [55]. The concern about an alcohol- or drug-impaired adult consenting for the care of a minor is that the parent may not be medically competent to do so. In these situations, it would be advisable to

postpone routine nonurgent medical care until consent can be obtained and to
clearly document in the medical record the reasons for delaying care [54]. In
emergency departments, this is less of an issue because the EMTALA statutes
clearly mandate that a medical screening evaluation must be performed whether
or not consent can be given. An additional concern in these cases stems from the
responsibility of all health care workers to report conditions of possible abuse and
danger to public safety. Clearly, the minor child of an alcohol- or drug-impaired
parent is at risk of maltreatment, but additional concerns must also include
allowing an impaired adult to drive a vehicle or administer medicines. Each state
has laws mandating that suspected child abuse and neglect must be reported, and
failure to do so can result in both criminal and civil penalties [54].

Refusal to care

In addition to issues related to consent for care, concerns over refusal of care
for children also arise. The Office of the United Nations High Commissioner for
Human Rights, Convention on the Rights of the Child assert: "In all actions
concerning children, whether undertaken by public or private social welfare
institutions, courts of law, administrative authorities or legislative bodies, the
best interests of the child shall be a primary consideration" [56]. The American
Academy of Pediatrics states: "Although physicians should seek parental permission in most situations, they must focus on the goal of providing appropriate care
and be prepared to seek legal intervention when parental refusal places the patient
at clear and substantial risk" [57].

The first step in resolving these situations is to improve communication between the health care providers and the parent or guardian. Often, when a physician simply listens to and addresses a parent's concerns and then slowly and
clearly explains the rationale for the desired intervention, an acceptable agreement can be made by both the physician and parent that will provide a high level
of care for a minor. Common reasons why parents do not consent to medical
treatment include anxiety and emotional turmoil, lack of education regarding a
procedure, poor physician-patient relationships, fears about technology, cost, loss
or absence from work, poor previous experiences, and religious or cultural
beliefs. In circumstances in which an agreement cannot be reached, a physician
has several options. If the intervention is not for an emergency condition, the
physician can provide the parents with information and have them return at a later
date to discuss the intervention; or the physician can allow the parent to request a
second opinion by another qualified physician; relent and agree to the parent's
wishes; remove themselves from the care of the child; or involve the child
protective services and legal systems to resolve the dilemma. No matter which
course is taken, the physician must ensure complete documentation of all discussions and plans. If the condition is an emergent or life-threatening condition,
the physician has a moral and ethical responsibility to provide the level of care
necessary to attempt to resolve the situation. In situations in which a consensus

cannot be reached and the physician believes that the patient is at significant risk without the proposed treatment, the physician may need to draw on other resources to help resolve the impasse [58]. However, it has been the present authors' experience that legal intervention is rarely necessary, especially when the most senior physician makes an honest effort to improve the communication between the health care professionals and the guardians of the minor.

Occasionally, a minor acting as an emancipated or mature minor may refuse to consent for treatment. Despite statutes and laws that protect the legal rights of minors to consent for care, most states have not addressed their right to refuse care [59], which is an even more complicated issue when the refusal of care will likely result in significant morbidity or mortality. The Patient Self Determination Act of 1990 mandated that health care providers and institutions provide their patients with written information about advance directives on hospital admission and that documentation of the advance directive must be documented in the medical record [60]. Unfortunately, the act does not require institutions to consider the legal rights or the decision-making capacity of emancipated or mature minors. The American Academy of Pediatrics has issued the following statement regarding life saving medical treatment (LSMT): "[P]hysicians and others should accord considerable weight to the feelings minor children may have expressed before losing the capacity to communicate clearly regarding LSMT. If the patient has executed a living will or any other form of advance directive for health care, that document should serve as strong evidence of the patient's wishes" [61].

Occasionally, a parent may refuse to consent for a minor's medical care on the basis of religious or cultural beliefs. Jehovah's Witnesses and Christian Scientists are the two most common religious doctrines that may dictate treatment refusal. Courts have consistently found that competent adults have the right to refuse medical treatment because they have a right to self-determination. As opposed to adults, children do not have a legal right to self-determination and rely on their parents to make decisions for their well being. Parental refusal of treatment for children on the basis of religious beliefs has been well documented in the literature, courts, and media.

The organization Children's Health Care is a Legal Duty reports over 200 deaths of children that have resulted from the refusal of medical care on the basis of religious beliefs [62]. Since the 1940s, the United States Supreme Court has held that "Parents may be free to become martyrs themselves, but it does not follow that they are free ... to make martyrs of their children before they reach the age of full and legal discretion when they can make that choice for themselves" [63]. In addition, the American Academy of Pediatrics believes that laws should not encourage or tolerate parental action that prevents implementing appropriate medical treatment, nor should laws exempt parents from criminal or civil liability in the name of religion [64]. Generally, physicians who seek court-mandated medical care for a child against the objections of parent are likely to succeed, particularly when the case calls for immediate intervention or when parental objections are religion based [65].

A wise statement by Dr. Kassuto addresses these dilemmas relating to consent: "Whenever there is a disagreement between the physician and the family, every effort should be made to find a compromise that would be acceptable to both parties. In situations where a consensus cannot be reached, and the physician feels that the patient is at significant risk without the proposed treatment, the physician may need to draw on other resources to help resolve the impasse. Nevertheless, careful consideration should be given before involving outside agencies, such as child protective services or the courts, because it has the potential of undermining the therapeutic relationship" [58].

Acknowledgments

The authors thank William J. Haynes III, Esq. for legal assistance.

References

[1] US Department of Health and Human Services, Centers for Medicare and Medicaid Services, Medicare Program. Clarifying policies related to the responsibilities of Medicare-participating hospitals in treating individuals with emergency medical conditions: final rule. 68 Federal Register 53222 (2003).
[2] Pub L No. 79–725, 42USC §§291 et seq.
[3] Rosenbaum S, Kamoie B. Finding a way through the hospital door: the role of emtala in public health emergencies. J Law Med Ethics 2003;31(4):590–601.
[4] Linzer JF. EMTALA: a clearer road in the future? Clin Ped Emerg Med 2003;4:249–55.
[5] Examination and treatment for emergency medical conditions and women in labor. 42 USC §1395dd.
[6] Special responsibilities of Medicare hospitals in emergency cases. 42 CFR 489.24(b).
[7] The Emergency Medical Labor and Treatment Act (EMTALA). Pub L No. 99–272, Title IX, [S]1395dd (1995), at [S] 1395dd9a.
[8] Li J, Galvin HK, Sandra JC. The "prudent layperson" definition of an emergency medical condition. Am J Emerg Med 2002;20(1):10.
[9] CFR §413,482,489. Fed Reg 2003;68(174):53,222–53,264.
[10] Glass DL, Rebstock J, Handberg E. Emergency Medical Treatment and Labor Act (EMTALA). Avoiding the pitfalls. J Perinat Neonatal Nurs 2004;18(2):103.
[11] McCaig LF, Burt CW. National Hospital Ambulatory Medical Care survey: 2003 emergency department summary. Advance data from vital and health statistics; no 358. Hyattsville (MD): National Center for Health Statistics; 2005.
[12] Carius M. Professional organizations in the emergency department. Emerg Med Clin North Am 2004;22(1):167.
[13] Fields WW, Asplin BR, Larkin GL, et al. The Emergency Medical Treatment and Labor Act as a federal health care safety net program. Acad Emerg Med 2001;8(11):1064.
[14] Jack N. Clinton unveils health reform. Los Angeles Times September 23, 1993:48.
[15] William RM. The cost of visits to emergency departments. N Engl J Med 1996;10:642.
[16] Simon HK, Ledbetter DA, Wright J. Societal savings by "fast tracking" lower acuity patients in an urban pediatric emergency department. Am J Emerg Med 1997;15:551.
[17] Reich WT. Oath of Hippocrates. In: Reich WT, editor. Encyclopedia of bioethics, volume 5. New York: Macmillan; 1995. p. 2632.

[18] Reich WT. World Medical Association, declaration of Geneva. In: Reich WT, editor. Encyclopedia of bioethics, volume 5. New York: Macmillan; 1995. p. 2646–7.

[19] American Medical Association. Principles of medical ethics. Available at www.ama-assn.org/ama/pub/category/2512.html or www.ama-assn.org. Accessed May 23, 2005.

[20] American College of Emergency Physicians. Code of ethics for emergency physicians 2004. Policy #400188. Available at www.acep.org/webportal/PracticeResources/PolicyStatementsByCategory/Ethics/CodeofEthicsforEmergencyPhysicians.htm or www.acep.org. Accessed May 23, 2005.

[21] Joint Commission on Accreditation of Healthcare Organizations. Setting the standard. Available at http://www.jcaho.org/general+public/patient+safety/setting_the_standard.pdf or www.jcaho.org. Accessed May 23, 2005.

[22] Moskop JC, Marco CA, Larkin GL, et al. From Hippocrates to HIPAA: privacy and confidentiality in emergency medicine: part I: conceptual, moral and legal foundations. Ann Emerg Med 2005;45(1):53–9.

[23] Scholastic, Inc. Scholastic Children's Dictionary. New York: Scholastic Inc; 2002. p. 113, 411.

[24] US Department of Health and Human Services, Office for Civil Rights. Summary of the HIPAA Privacy Rule. 2003; Office of the Federal Register. Available at www.hhs.gov/ocr/privacy summary.rtf; and www.hhs.gov/ocr/hipaa. Accessed May 23, 2005.

[25] American Academy of Pediatrics, Pediatric Practice Action Group and Task Force on Medical Informatics. Privacy protection of health information: patient rights and pediatrician responsibilities. Pediatrics 1999;104(4):973–7.

[26] Klein J, McNulty L, Flatau C. Teenager's self reported use of services and perceived access to confidential care. Arch Pediatr Adolesc Med 1998;152(7):676–82.

[27] Cheng TL, Savageau JA, Sattler AL, et al. Confidentiality in health care: a survey of knowledge, perceptions, and attitudes among high school students. JAMA 1993;269(11):1404–7.

[28] Hollander D. Some teenagers say they might not seek health care if they could not be assured of confidentiality. Fam Plann Perspect 1993;25(4):187.

[29] Ford CA, Millstein SG, Halpern-Felsher BL, et al. Influence of physician confidentiality assurances on adolescents' willingness to disclose information and seek future health care: a randomized controlled trial. JAMA 1997;278(12):1029–34.

[30] Ginsburg KR, Winn RJ, Rudy BJ, et al. How to reach sexual minority youth in the health care setting: the teens offer guidance. J Adolesc Health 2002;31(5):407–16.

[31] Reddy DM, Fleming R, Swain C. Effect of mandatory parental notification on adolescent girls' use of sexual health care services. JAMA 2002;288(6):710–4.

[32] Klein JD, Wilson KM, McNulty M, et al. Access to medical care for adolescents: results from the 1997 Commonwealth Fund Survey of the Health of Adolescent Girls. J Adolesc Health 1999;25(2):120–30.

[33] American Medical Association. American Medical Association code of ethics: confidential care for minors, 2002. Available at www.ama-assn.org/ama/pub/category/8355.html or www.ama-assn.org/. Accessed May 23, 2005.

[34] American Academy of Pediatrics, Committee on Adolescence. Contraception and adolescence. Pediatrics 1999;104(5):1161–6.

[35] American Academy of Family Physicians. American Academy of Family Physicians statement of policy on adolescent health care 2001. Available at www.aafp.org/x6613.xml or www.aafp.org. Accessed May 23, 2005.

[36] American College of Obstetricians and Gynecologists. Policies and materials on adolescent health of the American College of Obstetricians and Gynecologists. Available at www.acog.org/departments/dept_notice.cfm?recno=7&bulletin=3316 or www.acog.org. Accessed May 23, 2005.

[37] Ford C, English A, Sigman G. Confidential health care for adolescents: positional paper of the Society for Adolescent Medicine. J Adolesc Health 2004;35(2):160–7.

[38] US Department of Health and Human Services, Office for Civil Rights. Standards for privacy of individually identifiable health information. 2002. Available at www.hhs.gov/ocr/hipaa/final master.html or www.hhs.gov/ocr/hipaa. Accessed May 23, 2005.

[39] Mlinek EJ, Pierce J. Confidentiality and privacy breeches in a university hospital emergency department. Acad Emerg Med 1997;4(12):1142–6.

[40] Barlas D, Sama AE, Ward MF, et al. Comparison of the auditory and visual privacy of emergency department treatment areas with curtains versus those with solid walls. Ann Emerg Med 2001;38(2):135–9.

[41] Olsen JC, Sabin BR. Emergency department patient perceptions of privacy and confidentiality. J Emerg Med 2003;25(3):329–33.

[42] Knopp RK, Satterlee PA. Ethical issues in emergency medicine: confidentiality in the emergency department. Emerg Med Clin North Am 1999;17(2):385–96.

[43] Moskop JC, Marco CA, Larkin GL, et al. From Hippocrates to HIPAA: privacy and confidentiality in emergency medicine: part II: challenges in the emergency department. Ann Emerg Med 2005;45(1):60–7.

[44] Malcolm HA. Does privacy matter? former patients discuss their perceptions of privacy in shared hospital rooms. Nurs Ethics 2005;12(2):156–66.

[45] English A, Ford CA. The HIPAA privacy rule and adolescents: legal questions and clinical challenges. Perspect Sex Reprod Health 2004;36(2):80–6.

[46] Jones RK, Boonstra H. Confidential reproductive health services for minors: the potential impact of mandated parental involvement for contraception. Perspect Sex Reprod Health 2004; 36(5):182–91.

[47] American Academy of Pediatrics, Committee on Pediatric Emergency Medicine. Consent for medical services for children and adolescents. Pediatrics 1993;92(2):290–1.

[48] American Academy of Pediatrics, Committee on Pediatric Emergency Medicine. Consent for emergency medical services for children and adolescents. Pediatrics 2003;111(3):703–6.

[49] Treloa DJ, Peterson E, Randall J, et al. Use of emergency services by unaccompanied minors. Ann Emerg Med 1991;20(3):297–301.

[50] Bitterman RA. The medical screening examination requirement. In: Bitterman RA, editor. Providing emergency care under federal law: EMTALA: with new supplement. Dallas (TX): American College of Emergency Physicians; 2000. p. 23–65.

[51] Jacobstein CR, Baren JM. Ethical issues in emergency medicine: emergency department treatment of minors. Emerg Med Clin North Am 1999;17(2):341–52.

[52] Johnson JL, Leff M. Children of substance abusers: overview of research findings. Pediatrics 1999;103(5):1085–99.

[53] Grant BF. Estimates of US children exposed to alcohol abuse and dependence in the family. Am J Public Health 2000;90(1):112–5.

[54] Fraser JJ, McAbee GN. Dealing with the parent whose judgement is impaired by alcohol or drugs: legal and ethical considerations. Pediatrics 114(3):869–73.

[55] Berger JE. Consent by proxy for nonurgent pediatric care. Pediatrics 2003;112(5):1186–95.

[56] Office of the United Nations High Commissioner for Human Rights. Convention on the rights of the child 1989: part I: article 3. Available at www.unhchr.ch/html/menu3/b/k2crc.htm; and www.ohchr.org/english/bodies/crc/index.htm. Accessed May 23, 2005.

[57] American Academy of Pediatrics, Committee on Bioethics. Informed consent, parental permission, and assent in pediatric practice. Pediatrics 1995;95(2):314–7.

[58] Kassuto Z, Vaught W. Informed decision making and refusal of treatment. Clin Pediatr Emerg Med 2003;4(4):285–91.

[59] Zawistowski CA, Frader JE. Ethical problems in critical care: consent. Crit Care Med 2003; 31(5).

[60] Vaught W, Kassuto Z. Ethical challenges in the emergency care of adolescent patients. Clinical Pediatric Emergency Medicine 2003;4(1):69–74.

[61] American Academy of Pediatrics, Committee on Bioethics. Guidelines on forgoing life-sustaining medical treatment. Pediatrics 1994;93(3):532–6.

[62] Children's Healthcare. Children's healthcare is a legal duty. Data on injuries to children because of religion-based medical neglect, 2005. Available at www.childrenshealthcare.org. Accessed May 23, 2005.

[63] Linnard-Palmer L, Kools S. Parents' refusal of medical treatment based on religious and/or cultural beliefs: the law, ethical principles and clinical implications. J Pediatr Nurs 2004;19(5): 351–6.
[64] American Academy of Pediatrics, Committee on Bioethics. Religious exemptions from child abuse statutes. Pediatrics 1997;9(2):279–81.
[65] Derry R. Court-mediated disputes between physicians and families over the medical care of children. Arch Pediatr Adolesc Med 2004;158(9):891–6.

PEDIATRIC CLINICS
OF NORTH AMERICA

ELSEVIER
SAUNDERS

Pediatr Clin N Am 53 (2006) 157–165

Index

Note: Page numbers of article titles are in **boldface** type.

A

Abdominal injury, in child abuse, 34–35

Abdominal pain, **107–137**
  approach to, 107–109
  colic, 125–126
  extra-abdominal causes of, 107–109
  in appendicitis, 115–118
  in constipation, 113–115
  in gastroenteritis, 109–113
  in hypertrophic pyloric stenosis, 127–129
  in incarcerated hernia, 122–123
  in intestinal malrotation with volvulus,
    129–132
  in intussusception, 118–121
  in Meckel's diverticulum, 124–125
  in necrotizing enterocolitis, 132–133
  in small bowel obstruction, 121–122

Abuse, child. *See* Child abuse.

Abusive head trauma, 28–31, 72

Acromioclavicular joint, dislocations of, 45

Acyanotic heart disease, congenital, 81–82

Acyclovir
  for neonatal herpes, 75
  for neonatal sepsis, 75

Adenosine, for supraventricular tachycardia, 94

Adolescents, privacy rules concerning,
  146–147

Adrenal gland, congenital hyperplasia of, 81
  versus malrotation with midgut
    volvulus, 130

Air enema, for intussusception, 120

Alcohol intoxication, parental consent of care
  and, 149–150

Alkalosis, metabolic, in hypertrophic pyloric
  stenosis, 128

American Academy of Neurology
  concussion definition of, 3
  concussion grading scale of, 19–20

American Academy of Pediatrics
  mild head injury guidelines of, 13
  on life saving medical treatment, 151
  on refusal to care, 150

American Congress of Rehabilitation Medicine
  Head Injury Interdisciplinary Special Inter-
    est Group, mild head injury criteria of, 3

American Medical Association, ethical principles of, 144–145

Amiodarone
  for premature ventricular contractions, 90
  for supraventricular tachycardia, 94
  for tachycardias, 87
  for ventricular fibrillation, 91
  for ventricular tachycardia, 88–89

Ampicillin, for neonatal sepsis, 75

Angulation, of fractures, 45

Anterior humeral line, in fractures, 50

Antibiotics, for bacterial gastroenteritis, 113

Apparent life-threatening event, in neonates,
  72–73

Appendicitis, 115–118

Arrhythmias. *See* Dysrhythmias.

Arterial blood gas analysis, in cyanotic heart
  disease, 83

Atrial fibrillation, 96–97

Atrial flutter, 95–96

Atrial tachycardia, ectopic, 92–95

Atrioventricular block, 98–100

Atrioventricular nodal (junctional) tachycardia,
  92–95

Atrioventricular node reentrant tachycardia,
  92–95

Atropine
  for bradycardias, 97
  for hypertrophic pyloric stenosis, 129

Automated external defibrillators, for ventricular fibrillation, 91

Axillary nerve, injury of, in shoulder dislocation, 47

Axonal injury, in child abuse, 29

B

Barium enema, for intussusception, 120–121

Basilar skull fracture, 4

Behavior, after mild head injury, 16

Benzodiazepines, for seizures, 72

Beta-blockers
    for premature ventricular contractions, 90
    for prolonged QT syndrome, 103
    for supraventricular tachycardia, 94

Bicycle helmets, for head injury prevention, 2

Birth injuries
    brachial plexus palsy, 63–64
    clavicular fractures, 45–46
    humeral fractures, 47–48

Bisacodyl, for constipation, 114

Bleeding, rectal, in Meckel's diverticulum, 124–125

Bone scan, in child abuse, 30–31

Brachial plexus palsy, 63–64

Bradycardias
    causes of, 97
    conduction abnormalities, 98–100
    definition of, 97
    sinus, 97–98
    treatment of, 97

Brain
    injury of. *See also* Mild head injury.
        in child abuse, 28–31
        swelling of, in mild injury, 3

Breastfeeding
    rehydration techniques in, 112
    stool characteristics in, 113

Bronchiolitis, in neonates, 73–74

Bruises, in child abuse, 33–34

Bucket handle fractures, in child abuse, 31–32

Buckle fractures, 42, 60

Burns, in child abuse, 34

C

Campylobacter jejuni, in gastroenteritis, 113

Cantu concussion grading scale, 18–19

Cardiopulmonary resuscitation
    for bradycardias, 97
    for ventricular fibrillation, 91
    rib fracture risk in, 32

Cardioversion
    for atrial fibrillation, 97
    for supraventricular tachycardia, 94
    for tachycardias, 87
    for ventricular tachycardia, 88–89

Cefotaxime, for neonatal sepsis, 75

Child abuse, **27–39**
    abdominal injury in, 34–35
    cutaneous manifestations of, 33–34
    head trauma in, 28–31, 72
    medical provider role in, 27–28
    sexual, 35–37
    skeletal injury in, 31–32

Cigarette burns, in child abuse, 34

Clavicle
    dislocations of, 45–46
    fractures of, 45–46

Clostridium difficile, in gastroenteritis, 113

Cognitive function, after mild head injury, 16

Colic, 125–126

Colon, intussusception of, 118–121

Colorado Medical Society, concussion grading scale of, 19–20

Compartment syndrome, in supracondylar fracture, 52–53

Complete heart block, 99–100

Computed tomography
    in abusive head trauma, 30
    in appendicitis, 117
    in mild head injury, 9–12, 14

Concussion. *See* Mild head injury.

Conduction abnormalities, 98–100

Confidentiality, in EMTALA provisions, 144–147

Congenital adrenal hyperplasia, 81
    versus malrotation with midgut volvulus, 130

Congenital heart disorders
    atrial fibrillation in, 96
    atrial flutter in, 95
    in neonates, 81–83
    prolonged QT syndrome, 100–103

Congestive heart failure
    in congenital disorders, 81–82
    in tachycardia, 93–94

Consciousness, loss of, in mild head injury, 7

Consent of care, 147–152

Consolidated Omnibus Budget Reconciliation Act of 1985, EMTALA in. *See* Emergency Medical Treatment and Labor Act.

Constipation, 113–115

Corticosteroids, for bronchiolitis, 74

CRITOE acronym, in supracondylar fracture, 49

Crying, inconsolable, causes of, 126

Culture, stool, in gastroenteritis, 111

Currant jelly stool, in intussusception, 119

Cyanotic heart disease, congenital, 82–83

D

Defibrillation
    for tachycardias, 87
    for ventricular fibrillation, 91

Dehydration, in gastroenteritis, 110–113

Diabetic ketoacidosis, abdominal pain in, 111

Diarrhea
    in appendicitis, 116
    in gastroenteritis, 109–113

Diazepam, for seizures, 72

Diet, for constipation, 115

Digoxin, for atrial flutter, 96

Dinner fork deformity, in forearm fractures, 58–59

Dislocations
    clavicular, 45–46
    elbow, 54–56
    shoulder, 46–47
    wrist, 62

Displacement, of fractures, 44–45

Diverticulum, Meckel's, 124–125

Docusate, for constipation, 115

Doppler studies, in appendicitis, 117

"Double bubble" sign, in malrotation with midgut volvulus, 131

Ductus arteriosus, patent, 81–83

Dysrhythmias, **85–105**
    atrial fibrillation, 96–97
    atrial flutter, 95–96
    conduction abnormalities, 98–100
    electrocardiography in, 85–86. *See also specific dysrhythmias.*
    premature ventricular contractions, 89–90
    prolonged QT syndrome, 100–103
    sinus bradycardia, 97–98
    sinus tachycardia, 86, 88
    supraventricular tachycardia, 87, 91–95
    ventricular fibrillation, 87, 90–91
    ventricular tachycardia, 87–89

E

Ectopic atrial tachycardia, 92–95

Elbow
    dislocations of, 54–56
    fractures of
        lateral condylar, 53–54, 57
        medial condylar, 57
        medial epicondylar, 54
        olecranon, 56–57
        radial, 55–56
        supracondylar, 48–53
        transphyseal, 53
    nursemaid's, 57–58

Electrocardiography, 85–86. *See also specific dysrhythmias.*

Emergency Medical Treatment and Labor Act, **139–155**
    appropriate medical screening examination in, 142
    appropriate transfer in, 142–143
    clarifying policies for, 140–141
    confidentiality concerns in, 144–147
    consent of care in, 147–150
    controversies in, 143–144
    definition of, 140
    enactment of, 139–140
    new changes in, 141
    potential ambiguities in, 141
    privacy concerns in, 144–147
    refusal to care in, 150–152
    unchanged regulations in, 141

Emergency treatment
    Emergency Medical Treatment and Labor Act and, **139–155**
    of abdominal pain, **107–137**
    of child abuse, **27–39**
    of dysrhythmias, **85–105**
    of mild head injury, **1–26**
    of newborns, **69–84**
    of upper extremity injuries, **41–67**

EMTALA. *See* Emergency Medical treatment and Labor Act.

Endocrine emergencies, in neonates, 81

Enemas, for intussusception, 120–121

Enterocolitis, necrotizing, 76, 132–133

Epinephrine
  for bradycardias, 97
  for bronchiolitis, 74
  for tachycardias, 87

Erb-Duchenne-Klumpke palsy, 64

Erb's palsy, 64

Erythromycin, for bacterial gastroenteritis, 113

Escherichia coli, in gastroenteritis, 113

Ethics, of emergency care, 145

F

Fall(s)
    fractures in, 31
    head injury in, 2
    on an outstretched hand (FOOSH)
        elbow dislocation in, 55
        supracondylar fracture in, 48

Fat pads, in elbow injury, 49

Fecal impaction, 114–115

Felon, 63

Fingers, fractures of, 62

Fluid therapy
    for malrotation with midgut
        volvulus, 132
    for Meckel's diverticulum, 125

Forearm fractures, 58–61

Fractures
    clavicular, 45–46
    consultation on, 44–45
    displacement of, 44–45
    elbow, 55–57
        lateral condylar, 53–54, 57
        medial condylar, 57
        medial epicondylar, 54
        olecranon, 56–57
        supracondylar, 48–53
        transphyseal, 53
    evaluation of, 43
    finger, 61–62
    forearm, 58–61
    hand, 61–62
    humeral, 47–54
        at shoulder, 46
        lateral condylar, 53–54, 57
        medial condylar, 57
        medial epicondylar, 54
        supracondylar, 48–53
        T-condylar, 57
        transphyseal, 53
    imaging in, 44
    in adults versus children, 41–42

    in child abuse, 31–32
    olecranon, 56–57
    open, 44
    physeal, 41–43
    radial, 55–56, 58–61
    Salter-Harris, 42–43
    scapular, 46
    shoulder, 46
    skull, 3–4
    types of, 44–45
    ulnar, 58–61
    wrist, 61–62

Furosemide, for congestive heart failure, 82

G

Galeazzi fractures, 59–61

Gastroenteritis
    emergency treatment of, 109–113
    versus appendicitis, 116
    versus hypertrophic pyloric stenosis, 128
    versus intussusception, 119

Gastroesophageal reflux, versus hypertrophic
    pyloric stenosis, 128

Gastrointestinal emergencies, in neonates,
    76–77, 79

Genitourinary injuries, in sexual abuse, 35–37

Gentamicin, for neonatal sepsis, 75

Glasgow coma scores, in mild head injury, 6–7

Glenohumeral joint, dislocations of, 46–47

Greenstick fractures, 42
    forearm, 58, 60

Growth plates, injuries of, 41–43

H

Hand
    fractures of, 62
    infections of, 62–63

Head injury
    in child abuse, 28–31, 72
    in neonates, 72
    mild. *See* Mild head injury.

Health insurance, EMTALA and, 143–144

Health Insurance Portability and Accountabil-
    ity Act, Privacy Rule of, 145–147

Heart
    conduction abnormalities of, 98–100
    congenital disorders of. *See* Congenital
        heart disorders.
    dysrhythmias of. *See* Dysrhythmias.

Helmets, for head injury prevention, 2

Hematochezia, in small bowel obstruction, 121

Hematoma, scalp, in mild head injury, 7–8

Hemorrhage
  intracranial, in child abuse, 28–29
  retinal, in child abuse, 29–30
  subdural, in child abuse, 29

Hepatomegaly, in congenital heart
  disorders, 81

Hernia, incarcerated, 122–125, 128

Herpes simplex virus infections, in
  neonates, 75

Herpetic whitlow, 63

Hill-Burton Act, 139

HIPAA (Health Insurance Portability and
  Accountability Act), Privacy Rule of,
  145–147

Hirschsprung's disease
  toxic megacolon in, 76
  versus malrotation with midgut volvulus,
    130–131

Hospital Survey and Construction Act, 139

Humerus, fractures of, 47–54
  at birth, 47–48
  at shoulder, 46
  lateral condylar, 53–54, 57
  medial condylar, 57
  medial epicondylar, 54
  supracondylar, 48–53
  T-condylar, 57
  transphyseal, 53

Hydrocele, versus inguinal hernia, 123

Hyperbilirubinemia, neonatal, 77, 79

Hyperkalemia, in congenital adrenal
  hyperplasia, 81

Hyperoxia test, in cyanotic heart disease, 83

Hyperthyroidism, in neonates, 81

Hypertrophic pyloric stenosis, 127–130

Hypocalcemia, seizures in, 70

Hypoglycemia
  in congenital adrenal hyperplasia, 81
  seizures in, 70

Hyponatremia
  in congenital adrenal hyperplasia, 81
  seizures in, 70

Hypoxia
  in cyanotic heart disease, 82–83
  seizures in, 70

I

Inborn errors of metabolism, 78–80

Incarcerated hernia, 122–125, 128

Infant walkers, head injury due to, 2

Infections, in neonates, 74–75

Informed consent, 147–150

Inguinal hernia, incarcerated, 122–125, 128

Injury(ies)
  abdominal, in child abuse, 34–35
  birth. *See* Birth injuries.
  brain. *See also* Mild head injury.
    in child abuse, 28–31
  genitourinary, in sexual abuse, 35–37
  skeletal. *See also* Fractures.
    in child abuse, 31–32
  sports, 18–22
  upper extremity. *See* Upper
    extremity injuries.

Intussusception, 118–121, 128

J

Jaundice, neonatal, 77, 79

Jervell-Lange-Nielsen syndrome, 100–103

Joint Commission on Accreditation of Health
  Care Organizations, on privacy and confidentiality, 145

Junctional tachycardia, 92–95

K

Kanavel's signs, in tenosynovitis, 63

Ketoacidosis, diabetic, abdominal pain in, 111

Klumpke palsy, 64

L

Lactobacillus, for gastroenteritis, 113

Lactose intolerance, in gastroenteritis, 113

Lactulose, for constipation, 114–115

Ladd's bands, in malrotation with midgut volvulus, 129–130

Laxatives, for constipation, 114–115

Legal issues, in sexual abuse, 35

Leukocyte imaging, in appendicitis, 117

Lidocaine
  for premature ventricular contractions, 90
  for tachycardias, 87

for ventricular fibrillation, 91
for ventricular tachycardia, 88–89

Long QT syndrome, 100–103

Lorazepam, for seizures, 70, 72

Lugol's solution, for thyrotoxicosis, 81

Luxio erecta, 47

M

Magnesium
    for prolonged QT syndrome, 102
    for ventricular fibrillation, 91

Magnetic resonance imaging
    in abusive head trauma, 30
    in appendicitis, 117

Malrotation with midgut volvulus, 76, 129–132

Meckel's diverticulum, 124–125

Median nerve, injury of
    in elbow dislocation, 55
    in supracondylar fracture, 52

Megacolon, toxic, 76

Mental status, evaluation of, in mild head
    injury, 5

Metabolic alkalosis, in hypertrophic pyloric
    stenosis, 128

Metabolic emergencies, in neonates, 78–80

Metacarpal fractures, 62

Metaphyseal fractures
    forearm, 60
    in child abuse, 31–32

Metronidazole, for bacterial gastroenteritis, 113

Midazolam
    for seizures, 72
    for ventricular tachycardia, 88

Mild head injury, **1–26**, 14–17
    American Academy of Pediatrics guide-
        lines for, 13
    clinical indicators of, 4–8
    definition of, 3
    disposition of, 13–14
    epidemiology of, 1–2
    Glasgow coma scores in, 6–7
    imaging in, 11–12
    in children less than 2 years old, 8–11
    in falls, 2
    in sports, 18–22
    loss of consciousness in, 7
    mechanism of, 3
    outcome of, 14–17
    pathophysiology of, 2–4

primary, 3
scalp abnormalities in, 7–8
second impact syndrome in, 20–21
secondary, 3
seizures in, 14, 17–18

Milk of magnesia, for constipation, 114–115

Mineral oil, for constipation, 114–115

Minors
    consent of care for, 148–149, 151
    privacy rules concerning, 147

Mobitz heart blocks, 98–99

Monteggia fractures, 58–59

Motor vehicle accidents, head injury in, 2

N

Nadolol, for prolonged QT syndrome, 103

Nafcillin, for skin infections, 75

Nail injuries, 62

Necrotizing enterocolitis, 76, 132–133

Neonates, emergencies in, **69–84**
    brachial plexus palsy, 63–64
    cardiac, 81–83
    clavicular fractures, 45–46
    constipation, 113–115
    endocrine, 81
    gastrointestinal, 76–77, 79
    humeral fractures, 47–48
    hypertrophic pyloric stenosis, 127–128
    infectious, 74–75
    malrotation with midgut volvulus,
        129–132
    metabolic, 78–80
    necrotizing enterocolitis, 76, 132–133
    neurologic, 69–73
    respiratory, 73–74

Nerve injury, in supracondylar fracture, 52–53

Neurologic emergencies, in neonates, 69–73

Neurologic examination
    in mild head injury, 5
    in shoulder dislocation, 47

Neuropsychologic testing, of athletes, after
    mild head injury, 21–22

Nightstick injury, of forearm, 58

Norwalk virus, in gastroenteritis, 110

Nursemaid's elbow, 57–58

O

Obstipation, in small bowel obstruction, 121

Office of the United Nations High Commissioner for Human Rights, Convention on the Rights of the Child, on refusal to care, 150

Olecranon, fractures of, 56–57

"Olive," in hypertrophic pyloric stenosis, 127–128

Omphalitis, 75

Ondansetron, for gastroenteritis, 112

Oral rehydration, for gastroenteritis, 112

P

Pacemaker
 for atrioventricular block, 100
 for prolonged QT syndrome, 103

Pain, abdominal. *See* Abdominal pain.

Paronychia, 62–63

Patent ductus arteriosus, 81–83

Patient Self Determination Act of 1990, 151

Phalangeal fractures, 62

Phenobarbital, for seizures, 70, 72

Phenytoin, for seizures, 72

Phototherapy, for neonatal jaundice, 77

Physeal injuries, 41–43, 60

Ping-pong fractures, of skull, 4

Plastic deformity, of bone, 42, 58

Polyethylene glycol, for constipation, 114–115

Potassium, extracellular, in mild head injury, 3

Premature infants, necrotizing enterocolitis in, 132–133

Premature ventricular contractions, 89–90

Privacy, in EMTALA provisions, 144–147

Procainamide
 for premature ventricular contractions, 90
 for supraventricular tachycardia, 94
 for tachycardias, 87
 for ventricular tachycardia, 88–89

Prolonged QT syndrome, 100–103

Propranolol
 for atrial flutter, 96
 for prolonged QT syndrome, 103
 for thyrotoxicosis, 81

Propylthiouracil, for thyrotoxicosis, 81

Prostaglandins
 for cyanotic heart disease, 83
 for patent ductus arteriosus, 82

Psychosocial outcomes, after mild head injury, 16–17

Pulseless electrical activity, 87

Pyloric stenosis, hypertrophic, 127–130

Q

QT interval, prolonged, 100–103

R

Radial nerve, injury of, in supracondylar fracture, 52

Radiography
 in intussusception, 120–121
 in malrotation with midgut volvulus, 131
 in Meckel's diverticulum, 124–125
 in mild head injury, 11
 in shoulder dislocation, 47
 in small bowel obstruction, 122
 in supracondylar fracture, 49–50
 in upper extremity injuries, 44

Radionuclide studies, in appendicitis, 117

Radius
 fractures of, 55–56, 58–61
 subluxation of, 57–58

Rectal examination
 in abdominal pain, 109
 in intussusception, 119

Refusal to care, 150–152

Rehydration, for gastroenteritis, 112

Religious beliefs, refusal to consent of care and, 151

Respiratory emergencies, in neonates, 73–74

Resuscitation, in abdominal pain, 108–109

Retinal hemorrhage, in child abuse, 29–30

Rib fractures, in child abuse, 31–32

Romano-Ward syndrome, 100–103

R-on-T phenomenon, in premature ventricular contractions, 90

Rovsing's sign, in appendicitis, 115

S

Salmonella, in gastroenteritis, 113

Salter-Harris fracture classification, 42–43

Scalp, injury of, in mild head injury, 7–8

Scaphoid, fractures of, 61

Scapula, fractures of, 31–32, 46

Schoolwork, after mild head injury, 17

Second impact syndrome, in sports, 20–21

Seizures
    in mild head injury, 14, 17–18
    in neonates, 70–72

Senna, for constipation, 114

Separation, of fractures, 45

Sepsis, in neonates, 74–75

Sexual abuse, 35–37

Sexually transmitted infections, in child
    abuse, 37

Shaken baby syndrome, 28–31, 72

Shigella, in gastroenteritis, 113

Shock, in congenital adrenal hyperplasia, 81

Shoulder
    dislocations of, 46–47
    fractures of, 46

"Silk glove" sign, in inguinal hernia, 123

Sinus bradycardia, 97–98

Sinus tachycardia, 87, 89

Skin infections, in neonates, 75

Skull fractures, pathophysiology of, 3–4

Small intestine
    intussusception of, 118–121
    malrotation of, with midgut volvulus, 76,
      129–132
    Meckel's diverticulum of, 124–125
    obstruction of, 121–122

Sorbitol, for constipation, 114

Spanking, bruises in, 33

Sports injuries, concussions, 18–22

Sternal fractures, in child abuse, 31–32

Stool culture, in gastroenteritis, 111

Subdural hemorrhage, in child abuse, 29

Substance abuse, parental consent of care and,
    149–150

Sudden death, in prolonged QT syndrome, 101

Supracondylar fractures, 48–53

Supraventricular tachycardia, 87, 91–95

Syncope, in prolonged QT syndrome, 101

T

Tachycardias
    algorithm for, 87
    atrial, 91–97
    atrioventricular nodal (junctional), 92–95
    atrioventricular node reentrant, 92–95
    definition of, 86
    in congenital heart disorders, 81
    in prolonged QT syndrome, 100–103
    sinus, 87, 89
    supraventricular, 87, 91–95
    ventricular, 87–91

Tachypnea, in congenital heart disorders, 81

"Target" sign, in intussusception, 120

Technetium scans, in appendicitis, 117

Tenosynovitis, of hand, 63

Terrible Ts, for cyanotic heart disease, 82

THE MISFITS mnemonic, in neonatal neuro-
    logic disorders, 69–70

Thurston-Holland fragment, in lateral condyle
    fractures, 54

Thyrotoxicosis, in neonates, 81

Torsade de pointes, 101–102

Torus fractures, 42

Toxic megacolon, 76

Transfer, in EMTALA, 142–143

Trauma. *See* Injury(ies).

Trimethoprim-sulfamethoxazole, for bacterial
    gastroenteritis, 113

U

Ulna, fractures of, 58–61

Ulnar nerve, injury of
    in elbow dislocation, 55
    in supracondylar fracture, 52

Ultrasonography
    in appendicitis, 117
    in hypertrophic pyloric stenosis, 128–129
    in intussusception, 120
    in malrotation with midgut volvulus, 131

Umbilical hernia, incarcerated, 123–125

Upper extremity injuries, **41–67**
    brachial plexus palsy, 63–64
    clavicle, 45–46
    consultation on, 44–45
    elbow, 54–58
      dislocations, 54–56
      medial condylar, 57

olecranon fractures, 56–57
radial head and neck fractures,
　　55–56
radial head subluxation, 57–58
T-condylar fractures, 57
evaluation of, 43–44
forearm, 58–61
hand, 62–63
humerus, 47–54
　lateral condylar, 53–54, 57
　medial condylar, 57
　medial epicondylar, 54
　supracondylar, 48–53
　T-condylar, 57
　transphyseal, 53
imaging in, 44
physeal, 41–43
scapula, 46
shoulder, 46–47
versus adult injuries, 41–42
wrist, 61–62

Upper GI series
in hypertrophic pyloric stenosis, 129
in malrotation with midgut volvulus, 131

Urinalysis
in appendicitis, 116
in gastroenteritis, 111

Urinary tract infections, versus appendicitis, 116

V

Vagal maneuvers, for supraventricular tachy-
　cardia, 94

Vancomycin, for bacterial gastroenteritis, 113

Ventricular fibrillation, 87, 90–91

Ventricular tachycardia, 87–89

Volkmann's ischemic contracture, in compart-
　ment syndrome, 53

Volvulus
midgut, with malrotation, 76, 129–132
versus hypertrophic pyloric stenosis, 128

Vomiting
in appendicitis, 116
in gastroenteritis, 109–113
in hypertrophic pyloric stenosis, 127
in intussusception, 118–119
in malrotation with midgut volvulus, 130
in small bowel obstruction, 121–122

W

Walkers, infant, head injury due to, 2

Wenckebach heart block, 98–99

Whitlow, herpetic, 63

Wolff-Parkinson-White syndrome, 92–94

World Medical Association, on confidential-
　ity, 144

Wrist
dislocations of, 62
fractures of, 61–62

Y

Yogurt, for gastroenteritis, 113